SMALL MATTERS

MCGILL-QUEEN'S/ASSOCIATED MEDICAL SERVICES STUDIES IN THE HISTORY OF MEDICINE, HEALTH, AND SOCIETY

SERIES EDITORS: S.O. FREEDMAN AND J.T.H. CONNOR

Volumes in this series have financial support from Associated Medical Services, Inc. (AMS). Associated Medical Services Inc. was established in 1936 by Dr Jason Hannah as a pioneer prepaid not-for-profit health care organization in Ontario. With the advent of medicare, AMS became a charitable organization supporting innovations in academic medicine and health services, specifically the history of medicine and health care, as well as innovations in health professional education and bioethics.

1 Home Medicine
 The Newfoundland Experience
 John K. Crellin

2 A Long Way from Home
 The Tuberculosis Epidemic among the Inuit
 Pat Sandiford Grygier

3 Labrador Odyssey
 The Journal and Photographs of Eliot Curwen on the Second Voyage of Wilfred Grenfell, 1893
 Ronald Rompkey

4 Architecture in the Family Way
 Doctors, Houses, and Women, 1870–1900
 Annmarie Adams

5 Local Hospitals in Ancien Régime France
 Rationalization, Resistance, Renewal, 1530–1789
 Daniel Hickey

6 Foisted upon the Government?
 State Responsibilities, Family Obligations, and the Care of the Dependent Aged in Nineteenth-Century Ontario
 Edgar-André Montigny

7 A Young Man's Benefit
 The Independent Order of Odd Fellows and Sickness Insurance in the United States and Canada, 1860–1929
 George Emery and J.C. Herbert Emery

8 The Weariness, the Fever, and the Fret
 The Campaign against Tuberculosis in Canada, 1900–1950
 Katherine McCuaig

9 The War Diary of Clare Gass, 1915–1918
 Edited by Susan Mann

10 Committed to the State Asylum
 Insanity and Society in Nineteenth-Century Quebec and Ontario
 James E. Moran

11 Jessie Luther at the Grenfell Mission
 Edited by Ronald Rompkey

12 Negotiating Disease
 Power and Cancer Care, 1900–1950
 Barbara Clow

13 For Patients of Moderate Means
   *A Social History of the
   Voluntary Public General
   Hospital in Canada, 1890–1950*
   David Gagan and Rosemary
   Gagan

14 Into the House of Old
   *A History of Residential Care
   in British Columbia*
   Megan J. Davies

15 St Mary's
   *The History of a London
   Teaching Hospital*
   E.A. Heaman

16 Women, Health, and Nation
   *Canada and the United States
   since 1945*
   Edited by Georgina Feldberg,
   Molly Ladd-Taylor, Alison Li,
   and Kathryn McPherson

17 The Labrador Memoir of
   Dr Henry Paddon, 1912–1938
   Edited by Ronald Rompkey

18 J.B. Collip and the Development
   of Medical Research in Canada
   Extracts and Enterprise
   Alison Li

19 The Ontario Cancer Institute
   *Successes and Reverses at
   Sherbourne Street*
   E.A. McCulloch

20 Island Doctor
   *John Mackieson and Medicine in
   Nineteenth-Century Prince
   Edward Island*
   David A.E. Shephard

21 The Struggle to Serve
   *A History of the Moncton
   Hospital, 1895 to 1953*
   W.G. Godfrey

22 An Element of Hope
   *Radium and the Response to
   Cancer in Canada, 1900–1940*
   Charles Hayter

23 Labour in the Laboratory
   *Medical Laboratory Workers
   in the Maritimes, 1900–1950*
   Peter L. Twohig

24 Rockefeller Foundation Funding
   and Medical Education in
   Toronto, Montreal, and Halifax
   Marianne P. Fedunkiw

25 Push!
   *The Struggle for Midwifery
   in Ontario*
   Ivy Lynn Bourgeault

26 Mental Health and Canadian
   Society
   Historical Perspectives
   Edited by James Moran
   and David Wright

27 SARS in Context
   Memory, History, and Policy
   Edited by Jacalyn Duffin and
   Arthur Sweetman

28 Lyndhurst
   *Canada's First Rehabilitation
   Centre for People with Spinal
   Cord Injuries, 1945–1998*
   Geoffrey Reaume

29 J. Wendell Macleod
   Saskatchewan's "Red Dean"
   Louis Horlick

30 Who Killed the Queen?
   *The Story of a Community
   Hospital and How to Fix Public
   Health Care*
   Holly Dressel

31 Healing the World's Children
   *Interdisciplinary Perspectives on
   Health in the Twentieth Century*
   Edited by Cynthia Comacchio,
   Janet Golden, and George Weisz

32 A Canadian Surgeon in the
   Army of the Potomac
   Francis M. Wafer
   Edited by Cheryl A. Wells

33 A Sadly Troubled History
   *The Meanings of Suicide
   in the Modern Age*
   John Weaver

34 SARS Unmasked
   *Risk Communication of
   Pandemics and Influenza
   in Canada*
   Michael G. Tyshenko with assistance from Cathy Patterson

35 Tuberculosis Then and Now
   *Perspectives on the History
   of an Infectious Disease*
   Edited by Flurin Condrau
   and Michael Worboys

36 Caregiving on the Periphery
   *Historical Perspectives on
   Nursing and Midwifery in
   Canada*
   Edited by Myra Rutherdale

37 Infection of the Innocents
   *Wet Nurses, Infants, and
   Syphilis in France, 1780–1900*
   Joan Sherwood

38 The Fluorspar Mines of
   Newfoundland
   *Their History and the Epidemic
   of Radiation Lung Cancer*
   John R. Martin

39 Small Matters
   *Canadian Children in Sickness
   and Health, 1900–1940*
   Mona Gleason

Small Matters

Canadian Children in Sickness and Health, 1900–1940

MONA GLEASON

McGill-Queen's University Press
Montreal & Kingston • London • Ithaca

© McGill-Queen's University Press 2013

ISBN 978-0-7735-4132-0 (cloth)
ISBN 978-0-7735-4133-7 (paper)
ISBN 978-0-7735-8854-7 (ePDF)
ISBN 978-0-7735-8855-4 (ePUB)

Legal deposit second quarter 2013
Bibliothèque nationale du Québec

Printed in Canada on acid-free paper that is 100% ancient forest free (100% post-consumer recycled), processed chlorine free

This book has been published with the help of a grant from the Canadian Federation for the Humanities and Social Sciences, through the Awards to Scholarly Publications Program, using funds provided by the Social Sciences and Humanities Research Council of Canada.

McGill-Queen's University Press acknowledges the support of the Canada Council for the Arts for our publishing program. We also acknowledge the financial support of the Government of Canada through the Canada Book Fund for our publishing activities.

Library and Archives Canada Cataloguing in Publication

Gleason, Mona, 1964–
    Small matters: Canadian children in sickness and health, 1900-1940/ Mona Gleason.

    (McGill-Queen's/Associated Medical Services studies in the history of medicine, health and society, ISSN 1198-4503; 39)
    Includes bibliographical references and index.
    ISBN 978-0-7735-4132-0 (bound). – ISBN 978-0-7735-4133-7 (pbk.)
    ISBN 978-0-7735-8854-7 (ePDF). – ISBN 978-0-7735-8855-4 (ePUB)

    1. Children – Health and hygiene – Canada – History – 20th century. 2. Child health services – Canada – History – 20th century. 3. Physician and patient. 4. Pediatrics – Canada – History – 20th century. I. Title. II. Title: Canadian children in sickness and health, 1900-1940. III. Series: McGill-Queen's/Associated Medical Services studies in the history of medicine, health, and society; 39

    RJ103.C3G54 2013   613'.04320971   C2013-900117-4

This book was typeset by Interscript in 10.5/14 Sabon.

*For my parents, William (1923–1999)
and Margaret (1935–2012) Gleason*

Contents

Acknowledgments   xi

Illustrations   xv

Introduction: The Intimate Landscape of Health in the History of Children and Childhood   3

1 Doctored Bodies: Professional Medical Discourse and Children's Embodied Difference   21

2 Florence, Marc, Alice, and Theresa: Healthy Bodies and Domestic Doctoring, 1910s to the 1920s   46

3 Shirley, Lily, Jack, and Lina: Healthy Bodies and Domestic Doctoring, 1920s to the 1940s   67

4 Learning the Body: Schools, Curriculum, and Health   85

5 Treated Bodies: Hospitalization   102

6 Reforming the Body: Doctors, Educators, and Attitudes Towards Disability in Childhood   119

Conclusion: Small Matters: Historical Meaning and Children's Embodiment   138

APPENDICES

1 Causes of Infant Death in Canada   149

2 Participant Information   150

3 My Health Record   152

Notes 153

Selected Bibliography 187

Index 203

Acknowledgments

Health, our own and that of our loved ones, is a topic of endless discussion around dinner tables, at the local skating rink, in coffee shops, and across the neighbour's fence. It is a complex topic that interests all of us, links us together as human beings, and stretches across time. It is fitting that over the period I wrote this book about children's health experiences in the past, my own children endured various, though thankfully minor, childhood illnesses. Fever, scabies, infections, head lice, chicken pox – each, in turn, made their presence sorely felt. Sophie and Will took little comfort in the fact that their mother gained a little more historical insight and empathy each time they took to their beds or visited the doctor's office.

While I am the author of *Small Matters: Canadian Children in Sickness and Health, 1900–1940*, and solely responsible for errors and omissions, many people supported its completion. Funding provided by the Social Sciences and Humanities Research Council of Canada was critical to hire and train students, visit archives, gather documents, and conduct and transcribe oral history interviews. Co-operation on the part of librarians, archivists, and administrators of collections in Halifax, Toronto, Ottawa, Calgary, Vancouver, and Victoria was central to the research process. University of Toronto staff responsible for patient records at the Hospital for Sick Children, including Dr Lorelei Lingard and Dr Sarah Whyte, helpfully facilitated access to historical records. I am also grateful to Tony Diniz, executive director of the Child Development Institute, for permission to review records of the West End Crèche.

A number of fellow scholars generously read early drafts of chapters and offered invaluable advice and insight. Tamara Myers,

Veronica Strong-Boag, and Leslie Paris, colleagues at the University of British Columbia (UBC), deserve special mention for their unwavering (and patient) interest in my work. They also provided much personal support and affection as wonderful friends. Fellow faculty in the Department of Educational Studies (EDST) in the Faculty of Education at UBC also supported this project and I am fortunate to have such wonderful colleagues. Shermila Salgadoe, adminstrative manager in EDST deftly, and with good humour, kept track of the financial and other administrative aspects of the project. I am grateful to fellow historians who presented at the Lost Kids Workshop held at University of British Columbia in 2006, including Karen Dubinsky, Cynthia Comacchio, William Bush, Molly Ladd-Taylor, and Neil Sutherland for their excellent feedback on ideas carried forward in this book. Likewise, the opportunity to share this research with fellow scholars at the Peter Wall Institute for Advanced Studies through the Early Career (Associate Level) Scholars Program at UBC in 2007–08 provided stimulating cross-disciplinary discussions of children and health. Fellow members of the Canadian History of Education Association, History of Children and Youth Group and the Society for the History of Children and Youth were, and are, a constant source of inspiration regarding the rich possibilities of work in the field.

I was fortunate to have excellent researchers work on this project. Graduate students, including Shaista Patel, Satnam Chahal, Lori MacFadyen, Natalie Chambers, Michelle Swann, Rose Ellis, Kristen Greene, Jessie Sutherland, Anthony Meza-Wilson, Anika Stafford, and Yesman Post, helped gather records and inputted data for analysis. Natalie and Lori conducted and transcribed most of the oral history interviews that form the backbone of the work. The women and men interviewed deserve a special thank you for their willingness to share their valuable experiences. Although their identities are protected by anonymity, without them this book would not have been possible. Margot Smythe was generous with her expertise on public health issues related to contemporary children and I very much valued our conversations and her interest in the work. Jacqueline Mason, Ryan Van Huijstee, and everyone at McGill-Queen's University Press provided excellent advice and assistance. I am grateful also to the editing suggestions of Jennifer Charlton and the anonymous readers of the manuscript who offered generous and insightful critique.

I am fortunate to have a loving circle of family and friends who encouraged me to live my life despite the constant work and worry associated with writing a book. Melinda Friedman, Marian De Gier, Myriam Brulot, Suzanne Smythe, Tess Prendergast, the ladies of the Glen Park Book Club, and neighbours in Vancouver's Cedar Cottage provided the perfect mix of sustenance and joyful respite from work. Grant and Gordon Bragg always maintained an interest in my writing and consistently offered their support. My parents, William and Margaret Gleason, supplied the priceless gift of unconditional love over their lifetimes. I will miss them every day. My sisters, Lynda Monteith and Margot Brown, were certain that I would succeed even as I doubted myself. Over the many years it took to finish the project, Sophie and Will kept me grounded and reminded me what my real job was. In the process, they made me a better historian. Finally, for saving my life, I owe my beloved Eric Roberts a debt that can never truly be repaid.

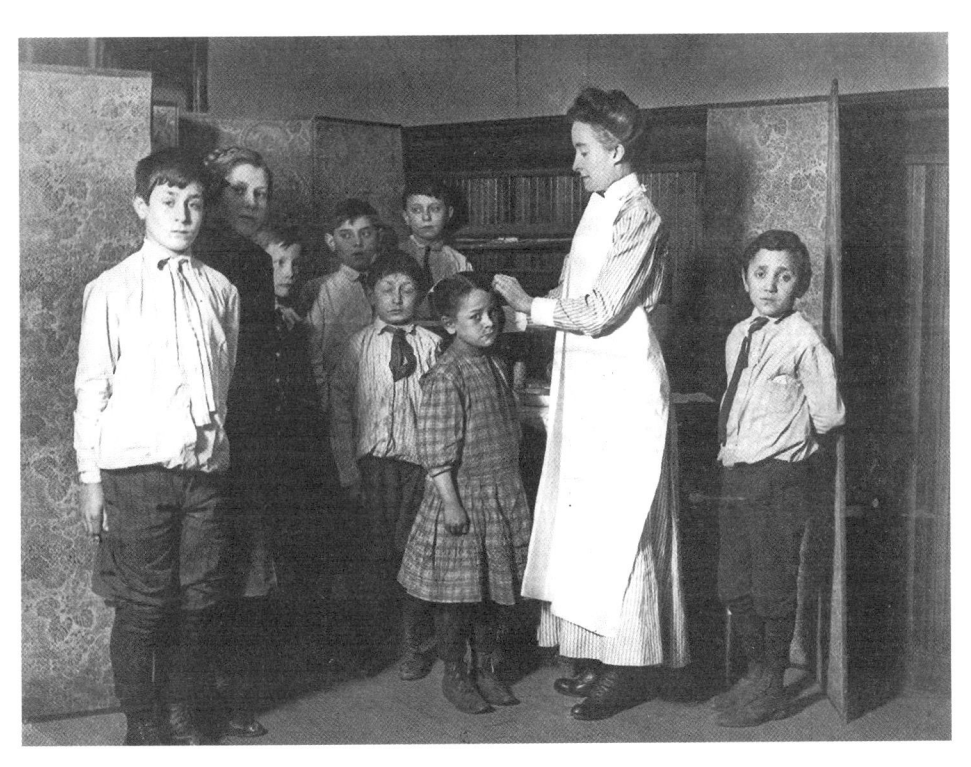

Children being washed by a nurse at school, 1905.
RG 10-30-2, 3.03.4, Archives of Ontario

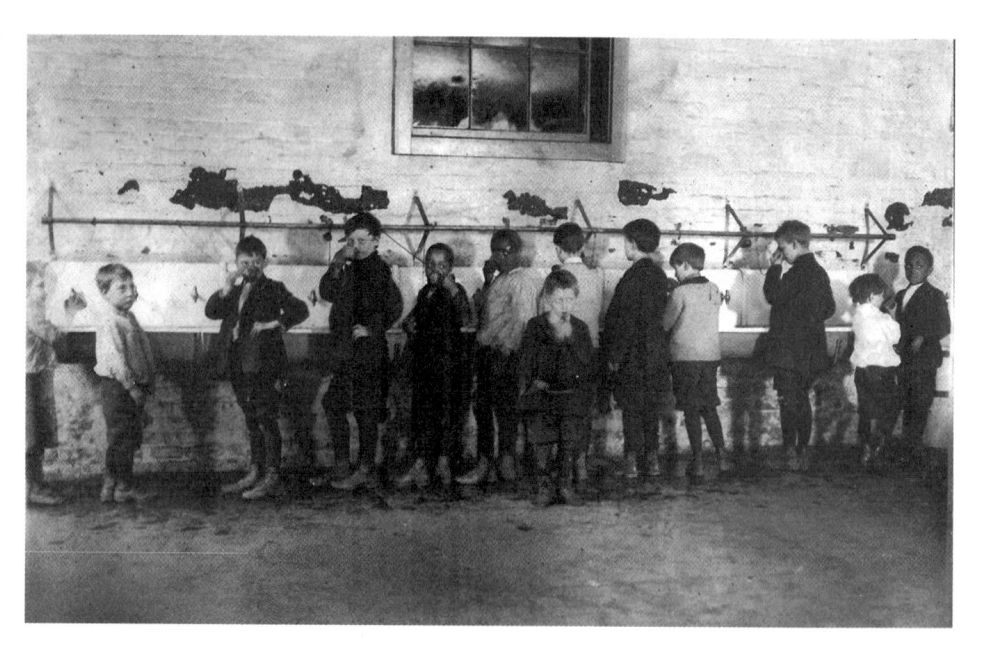

Children using unsanitary drinking cups, 1905.
RG 10-30-2, 3.03.6, Archives of Ontario

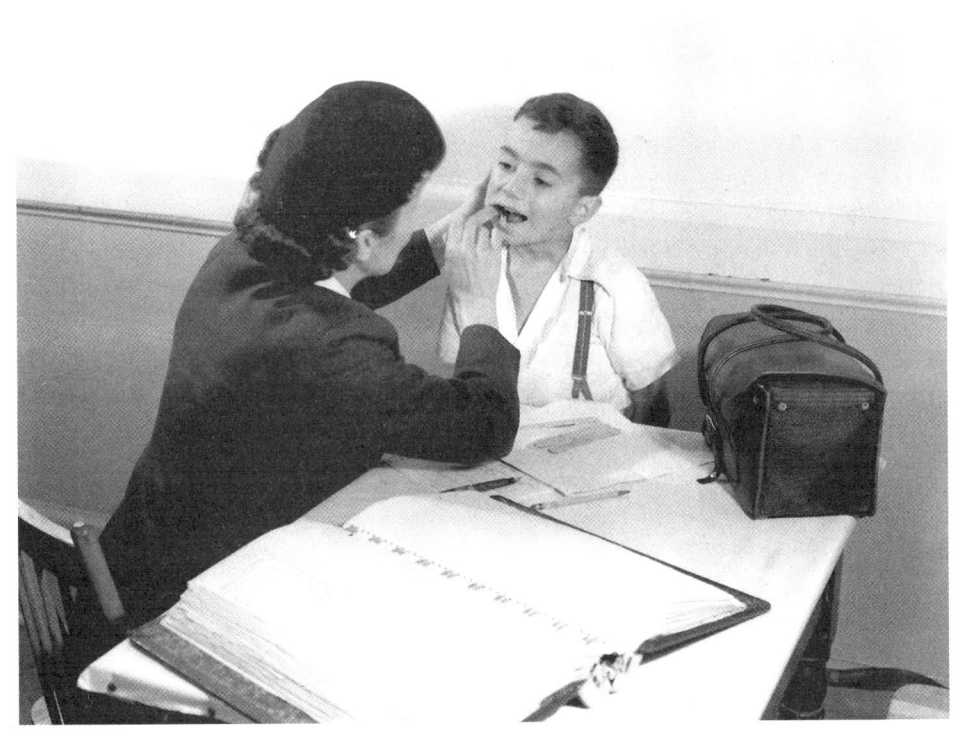

School health services nurse examining child's mouth, 1949.
I-00376, Royal BC Museum, BC Archives

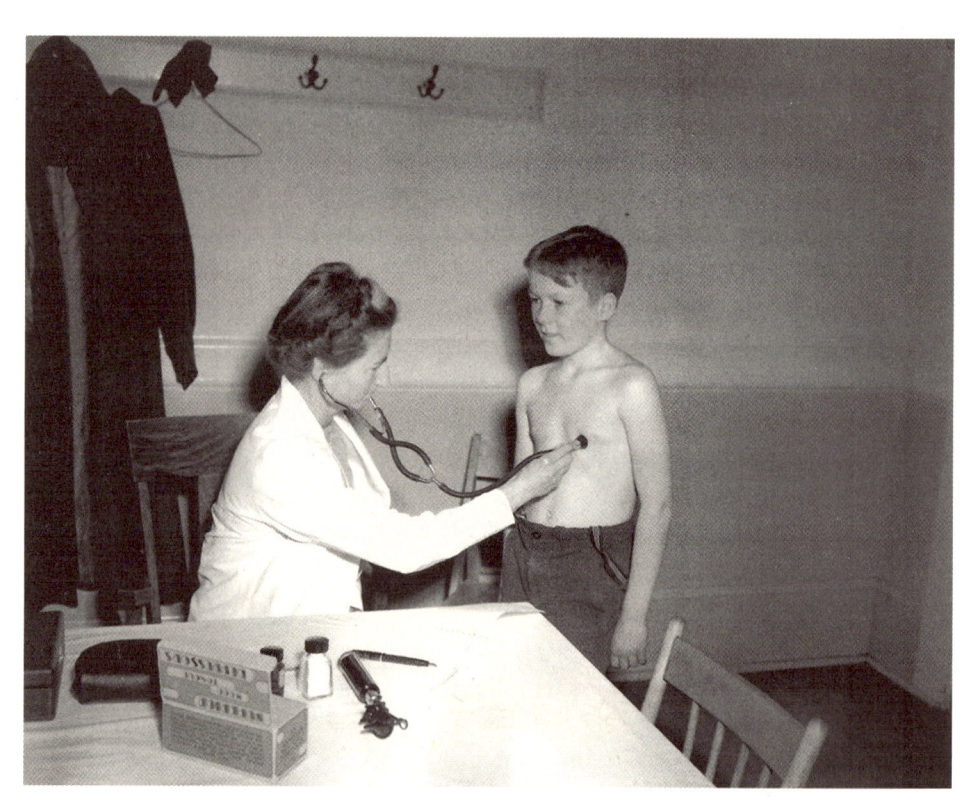

School health services nurse using stethoscope, 1949.
I-00377, Royal BC Museum, BC Archives

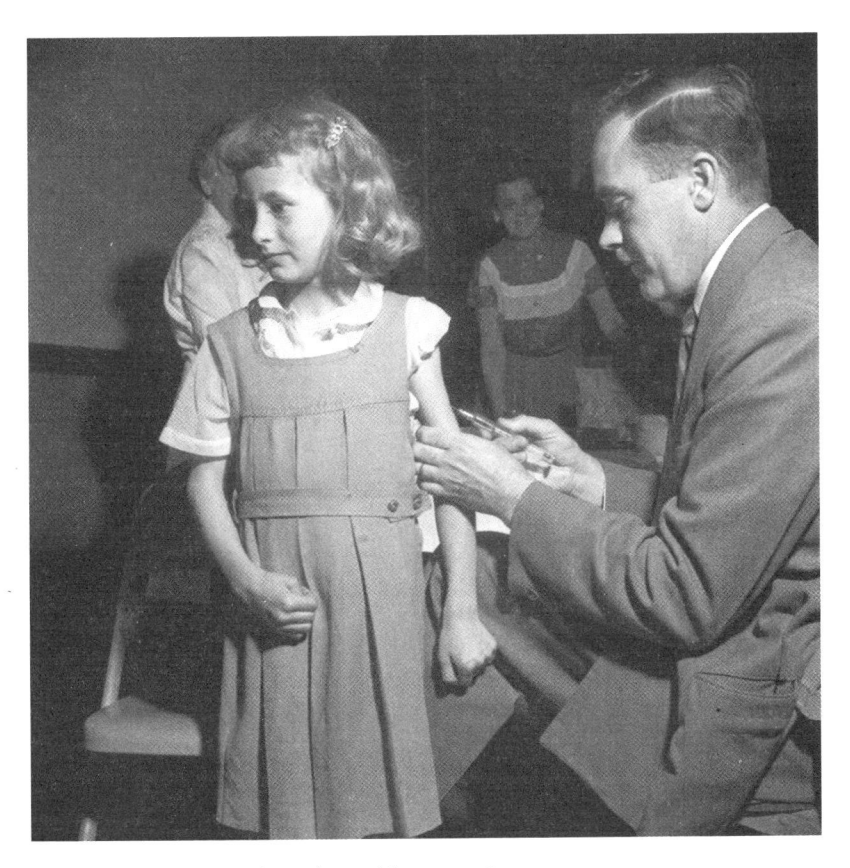

Polio injections in schools, Calgary, Alberta, 18 June 1954.
NA-5600-7434c, Glenbow Archives

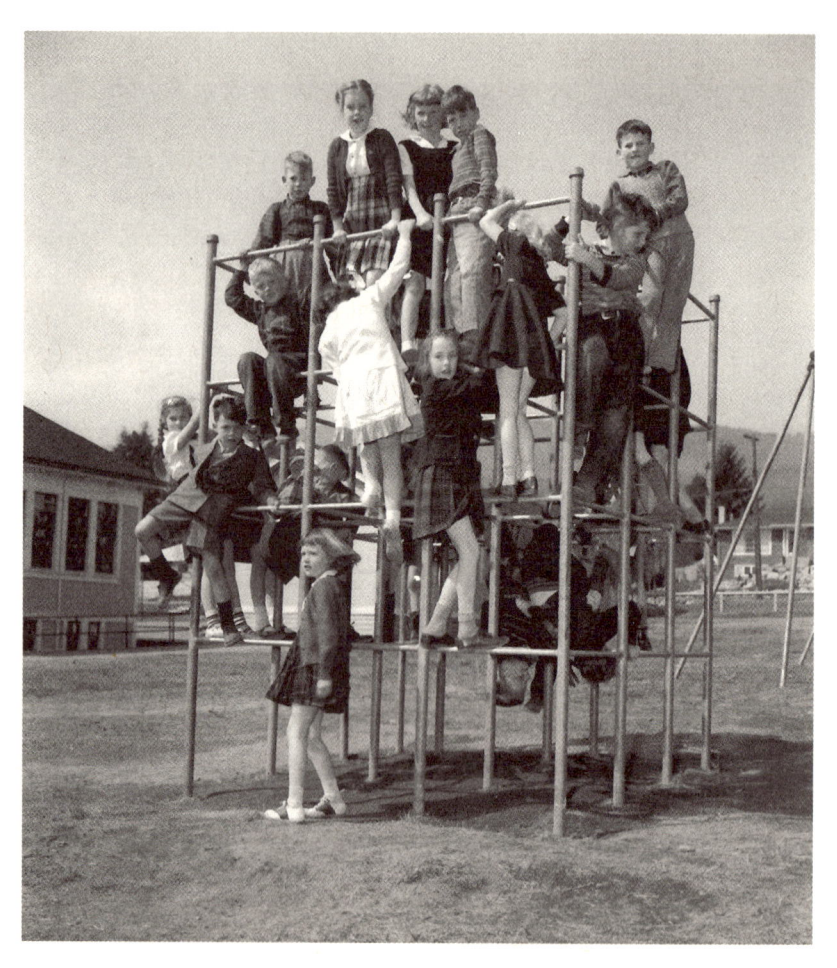

School children playing on jungle gym at Hollyburn Elementary School, 1950.
81256C, Vancouver Public Library

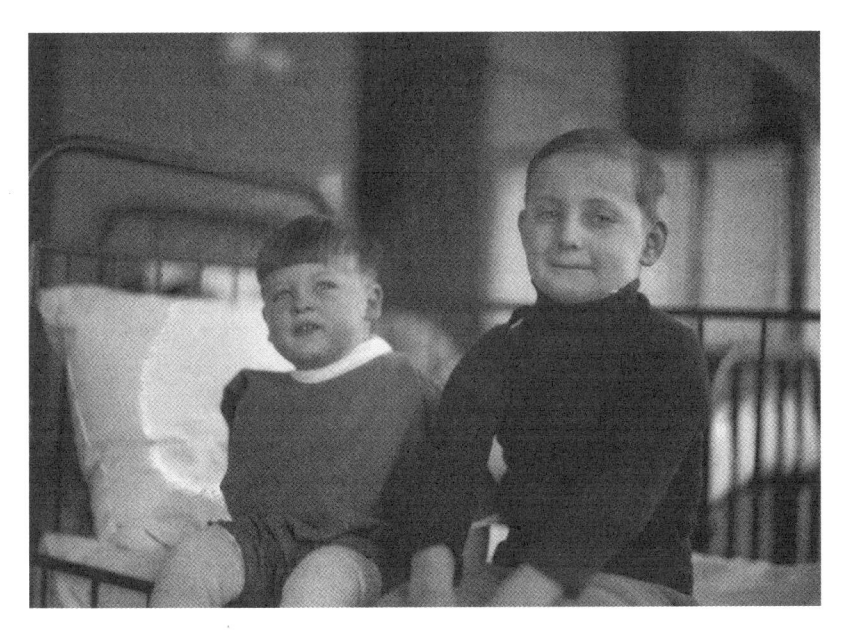

Children at Red Cross Hospital, Edmonton, Alberta, January 1928.
NC-6-12146d, Glenbow Archives

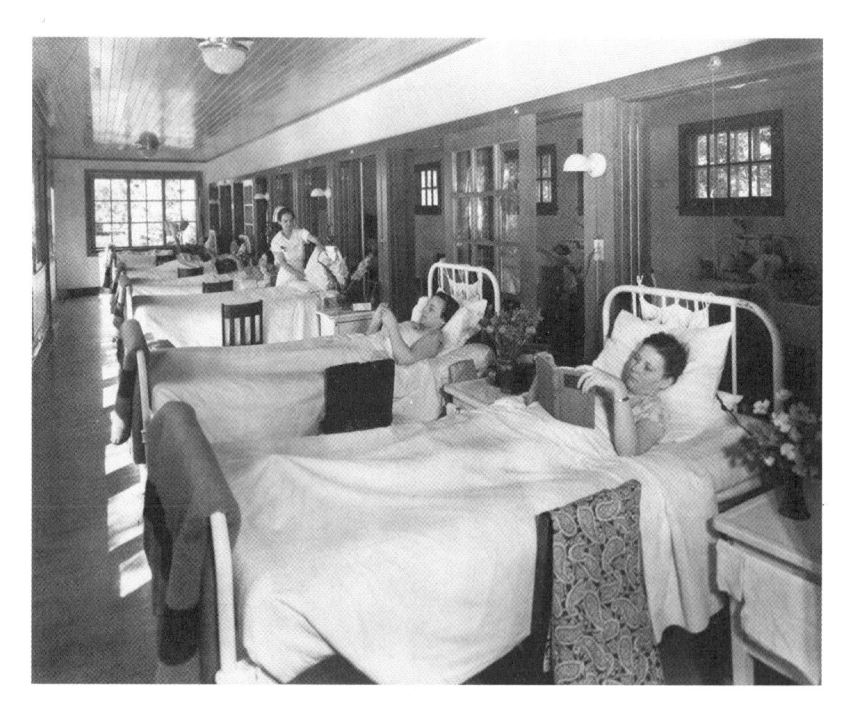

Patient ward, Central Alberta Sanatorium, Keith District, Calgary, Alberta, ca. 1927–1929.
NA-2910-18, Glenbow Archives

SMALL MATTERS

INTRODUCTION

The Intimate Landscape of Health in the History of Children and Childhood

Mattie Clarke was three years old in 1916. Born in Winnipeg, she had three siblings and lived in a modest house with her father, employed as a barber, and her mother, who tended to home and children full time. Once a week, her mother took her to the Children's Hospital to tend to a throat ailment. "There was something wrong with my throat," she recalled, "but I don't remember what they did to fix it." During her visit, Mattie would be "knocked out" by anesthesia, treated, and carried back home by her mother. "She would have to carry me from the streetcar, which was a great long block, and I'm sure she must have been exhausted since I wasn't a little skinny kid, I was a fat kid!" When the deadly influenza pandemic of 1918 hit the city, Mattie was five years old. She remembered that it killed many people in the city, but her family was spared much first hand experience. "We didn't have any time to be sick," Mattie recalled.[1]

In 1935, eleven-year-old Catherine Tilley, born in Bing Inlet, Ontario to a family of eleven children, suffered a high fever caused by measles. She dreaded going to sleep during her illness.

> As soon as I would close my eyes it was like black clouds of booming thunder that would roll in on me ... and then I remember being in the bed ... I was hallucinating I guess, and ... I got out of bed and I went running downstairs and Sarah, my sister, was down there with Mom and I was fighting them. I said, "I saw you fighting, I saw you fighting!" And

they told me this afterwards and I guess I was really out of my head with fever.[2]

Megumi Itou was born in Ocean Falls, British Columbia in 1941. Evacuated to Iron Springs, Alberta with other Canadians of Japanese descent during the Second World War, Megumi remembers "growing up poor" after her family's assets were taken away by government order. Along with around twenty-five hundred former residents of Ocean Falls, the Itous were forced to begin their lives again. Her father did farm labour and her mother remained at home, in charge of Megumi and her five siblings. Megumi's mother was also in charge of ensuring that, as much as possible, illness was avoided. To this end, she prepared many tonics and other home remedies to ward off illness. Hot lemonade, made with lemon peels, soothed cold symptoms and was a good source of vitamin C. Megumi remembered begging her mother to add sugar or honey to the lemonade, taming the sour taste and turning it into a welcome treat. When more serious illness occurred, Megumi remembered that she had to eat pickled garlic. "If the pickled garlic came out," she recalled, "I knew I had to get better very quickly."[3]

John Brennan was born in 1942 in North York, Ontario and contracted polio when he was five years old. He was hospitalized for two months at Toronto's Hospital for Sick Children (HSC) and then spent six months in a wheelchair. Two aspects of this experience stand out in his memory: his complete isolation from his family during his hospitalization and the painful injections he had to endure. "I remember getting the big needle. It seemed like it was six miles long at the time," he recalled. While walking to choir practice several years after he had recovered much of his mobility, John was hit by a car. He was hospitalized again, but only for three days. "I guess they were just watching me more than anything else," he reasoned, "because I didn't break any bones or anything. I guess they were watching for internal injuries or something." John remembered that "they had to call another ambulance to the accident scene because the first one was driven by my dad."[4]

The memories of Mattie, Catherine, Megumi, and John suggest the important place that health and the body – burdensome bodies, fevered bodies, sick bodies, injured bodies – occupy in memories of growing up.[5] Excerpted from longer oral history interviews, the memories give us some sense of what it felt like to be sick as a child in the past. They speak to the central place that context, home, and family played when illness or injury struck, how fear and apprehension could accompany professional medical treatment, and how such treatment was far from uniformly experienced or even uniformly relevant. In other oral histories included in this book, adults recall time spent in hospital or in bed with fever, serious injuries, or encounters with death and disease; the varying degrees of success associated with medicines handed over by doctors or concocted in kitchens; and lessons in school about proper nose-blowing or inoculations in the school gymnasium. Amidst the unique richness of each individual story of growing up, the intertwined centrality of home, family, and the body – especially in memories involving health and illness – marks a common theme.

Concern for the cultivation and provision of good health has long engaged Canadians in their homes, schools, and on various political stages: national, provincial, and local. Over the course of the twentieth century, the welfare state in Canada emerged in the shadow of liberal ideals of individualism and gendered notions of citizenship and entitlement linked primarily to adult males.[6] As Veronica Strong-Boag has shown, the "helping professions" of social work, teaching, and nursing/medicine helped foster the growth of state-sponsored welfare services, including health services, but did so in the midst of two often competing ideas: those that "stressed individual responsibility and those that emphasized the structural problems of unemployment and poverty."[7] Enveloped within these individual and structural approaches to social need, adult reformers, represented variously by religious authorities, philanthropists, social workers, educators, governmental officials, doctors, nurses, judges, lawyers, police officers, truant officers, psychologists, psychiatrists, and others, vied for authority in the lives of children and their families.[8] The growth and development of medical expertise, public health, and sanitation services in the late nineteenth century spawned demands in the twentieth for increased state involvement in the provision of a national health system. These calls became increasingly shrill in the years of the Great Depression when even the most recalcitrant defenders of the status quo – doctors – craved the stability that such a system promised. The financial investment needed to mount and defend a national system of health insurance, however, was judged unattainable in the lean 1930s. A number of attempts on the part of the provinces, namely Alberta and British Columbia, to enact a provincial health insurance system in the mid-1930s failed. Prime Minister William Lyon Mackenzie King's promise to introduce a national program was not forthcoming. Not until 1944, after over a decade of wrangling over jurisdiction and financial responsibilities, would the Department of National Health and Welfare be in place. Another two decades, similarly marked by contestation over cost sharing between the federal and provincial governments, would pass before Prime Minister Lester Pearson introduced the *Medical Care Insurance Act* in 1966.[9]

A number of studies in the North American context have considered more specifically the role of infants, children, and adolescents in broader histories of public health and welfare reform,[10] medical professionalization and specialization,[11] the evolution of children's hospitals,[12] and treatment protocols for particular health challenges associated with youngsters over the early decades of the twentieth century.[13] Less understood, most particularly in the Canadian context, is the everyday engagement with sickness and health that shaped the lives of the young and their families. Some important work has nonetheless begun to clear a new path of understanding. In her fine history of tragedy, resilience, and resistance in Winnipeg's response to the 1918 influenza pandemic, Esyllt Jones interprets the significance of the disease through the perspective of families, workers, fathers, mothers, volunteers, professionals, and children. She lays bare the pivotal difference that gender, race, class, and age made to the intimate experience of an influenza that lasted just over a year and killed approximately fifty-five thousand Canadians.[14] My book broadens this new path, placing childhood memories of experiences with health professionals, health imperatives, and a range of other health-related issues from the early 1900s to the 1940s in Canada at the heart of analysis and interpretation. The growth of the welfare state and the politics of ensuring healthy Canadians has long been a scholarly focus because, as Denise Gastaldo suggests, "in this century, health has become increasingly important politically as a major point of contact between government and population."[15] However, what this "point of contact" meant in the lives and on the bodies of youngsters who were so often the targets of health and welfare reform remains relatively unexplored. Three key questions posed in this book give some insight into this intimate landscape: how did medical and educational professionals understand the health needs and bodies of children and how did this change over the early decades of the twentieth century? What did the physical body mean in the context of a healthy childhood to children themselves and their families? What are we to make of the confluences and divergences in these perspectives and experiences?

While state-sponsored health and welfare reform in the twentieth century marked a considerable shift from the nineteenth century's focus on philanthropic and institutional approaches, youngsters and their families were constant targets of these efforts. The establishment of charitable orphanages, foundling homes, and children's hospitals in the West in the nineteenth century aimed to affect the moral reform of the "destitute classes," but it was through the containment and reformation of small and young bodies that this was believed best achieved.[16] In their foundational history of efforts to rescue and reform destitute children in nineteenth century Canada, Patricia Rooke and R.L. Schnell demonstrate how such efforts were justified and motivated by the new ideology of childhood evident in the West by the end of the seventeenth century.[17] The protection and improvement of children's lives exemplified long-evolving attitudes towards childhood as a time separate from the worries, strains, and obligations associated with adulthood.[18] Childhood, the new ideology suggested, was a time of dependence, protection, segregation, and delayed responsibility.[19] It was a period set aside for education, cultivation, and, as Viviana Zelizer has argued, the "sentimentalization" of the young.[20] Qualities associated with children in this new conceptualization of a protected and segregated childhood, such as innocence, vulnerability, incompetence, and unpredictability, guided and legitimized the work of twentieth-century reformers, defined the essence of children's "nature," and characterized qualities of their physical bodies. Given their social and professional authority over matters of the body, medical practitioners – doctors in particular, but also nurses – and educators, especially teachers, took up and entrenched views of children as requiring considerable protection, discipline, surveillance, and guidance.[21]

Scholarship in the social history of Canada, and indeed North America and Europe, has provided a solid foundation for our understanding of the perspectives of professional adults on the meaning of a "proper childhood." A number of historians have been careful to point out that twentieth century welfare reform was never an entirely positive force for all youngsters. Critical studies in various national contexts have placed health and welfare initiatives into conversation with broader social, regional, cultural, and intellectual change, laying bare the political and ideological interests of socially powerful adults conveyed through child-saving.[22] Those whose race, gender, class, or disability set them apart from the white, Anglo-Protestant, middle-class "norm" tended to bear the brunt of interventionist practices and discourses emanating from reformers. Nic Clarke has shown how, in the case of children with intellectual disabilities in British Columbia in the early twentieth century, sentimentalization did not always apply to those so often "demonized" as a burden on the state.[23] In Quebec, Catholicism profoundly shaped the tenor of child-saving. "If the problem of child protection is of prime importance economically, nationally, and socially speaking," argued Abbé Charles E. Bourgeois in 1948, "its religious aspect surely prevails over all others ... the religious and supernatural training of dependent children is undoubtedly, all-important."[24] As Denyse Baillargeon has shown in her history of maternal health in Quebec, the triad of the state, the clergy, and the medical profession joined forces to combat high rates of infant and maternal mortality at the turn of the century. As long as the services offered by each were complimentary and did not threaten the status quo, the balance between the forces of nationalism, Catholicism, and saving lives satisfied the triad. However, when the balance was threatened, consensus broke down. The increased involvement of municipal layers of government in infant health in Montreal was, for example, seen as a threat to the parish-controlled *Goutte de lait* movement established early in the new century. Such wrangling between the provision of parish services and municipal services continued over the century causing what Baillargeon characterized as "bitter struggles" in the race to control the untimely deaths of mothers and babies.[25]

Concern for the health of young people nevertheless proved a common focus across the country in the new century. As much as this represented an investment in the emergent "dominion of youth," as Cynthia Comacchio's groundbreaking history on adolescence in Canada has shown, the provision of healthy children justified the work of professional adults in a number of circles, including government, medicine, social welfare, juvenile justice, religious orders, and education.[26] Late nineteenth-century compulsory school and child labour laws, despite their considerable limitations, signaled changing attitudes towards proper undertakings for youthful bodies.[27] These laws and other action on the part of the state, such as compulsory vaccination, water fluoridation, school medical inspection, and the interventions of juvenile courts, however beneficial for some, did not go uncontested by unwilling children and parents.[28] The imposition and enforcement of these laws and procedures nevertheless suggests the degree to which concerns about children's health status were braided with protection, disciplinary, and dependency-oriented views of childhood.

In concert with these efforts, educational professionals wrote dominant ideas of health and healthy living into school curricula. Compulsory schooling promised that increasing numbers of children attended schools for longer periods of time, particularly in urban settings.[29] To an increasingly captive audience, schools communicated social standards of cleanliness, disease eradication, and prevention directly to Canadian families through their children. Little wonder then that schools were quickly seized upon as critical sites for the dissemination of information. As early as the turn of the century, some educators stressed how bothersome this had already become. Agnes Deans Cameron, principal of South Park School in Victoria, British Columbia complained in 1900 that schools had become "tempting fields easy of access to every hobby-horse rider for the introduction of what each considers the sine qua non for reforming the world."[30] Despite such concerns, schools, at least rhetorically, aspired to be perfect "health laboratories" where large numbers of young people could be taught about health standards, placed under surveillance, measured, examined, vaccinated, and even operated upon. Official health curriculum early in the twentieth century linked the observance of "good habits of health" with Christian morality and white, middle-class citizenship. Over the course of the century, health curriculum would shift again to reflect new emphasis on "democratic citizenship."[31] Protecting and improving children by segregating, training, treating, and improving their bodies represented a major component of the developing social welfare apparatus in North America and the West more generally in the twentieth century, and reflected new thinking about the constitution of "childhood."

From the perspective of children and their families, medical and educational health interventions had mixed consequences. In the chapters that follow, the complexities of these relationships are explored from various perspectives. Constraints based on race, class, gender, sexuality, and ability played a significant role in determining who benefited from professional attention and who did not. The desire for positive improvements to children's health that justified many medical and educational interventions could, and sometimes did, have the opposite outcome. Habits and bodies judged "healthy" by authorities did not always match up easily, or at all, with the realities, capacities, or priorities of young people and their families. This proved to be a considerable burden for some. Mandatory attendance at public schools, a major tenet of health and welfare reform, for example, could itself have deleterious effects on health: public schools were crowded, often unhealthy spaces for children in which contagions of all manner spread quickly through the attending population.[32]

Nevertheless, medical and educational professionals worked diligently to reinforce the message that pathologies that accompanied being young and small could be confronted and bested. By the 1920s and 1930s, health and welfare interventions shifted from concern over levels of maternal and infant death, to control of contagious diseases and the promotion of vaccination, to the prevention of disease and accidental death.[33] The automobile and consumer products poisonous to youngsters, in particular, were deadly developments for children. One in every six persons killed in an automobile accident in 1934, for example, was a child under fifteen years of age.

This figure continued to rise well past the Second World War.[34] By 1997, 963 Canadians under the age of nineteen died from accidental injury.[35] The child mortality rate attributed to suicide has increased two-an-a-half times, from three deaths per million in 1971 to eight deaths per million in 1996.[36] In 2002, suicide accounted for 24 per cent of all deaths among fifteen– to twenty–four–year–olds and was the second leading cause of death for Canadians between the ages of ten and twenty-four years.[37] While adults, particularly white, middle-class adults, rarely acknowledged the role they played in *creating* some aspects of children's vulnerability to ill health and mortality, they were nevertheless increasingly clear about how to prevent it or at least manage its affects.

It is crucial to acknowledge, however, that the intervention of middle-class reformers was never simply negative for children and their families. As Neil Sutherland demonstrated in his foundational study of the growth of public health reform aimed at Canadian children over the twentieth century, efforts to reduce high rates of infant mortality and, by the 1920s, to control killer contagions, such as whooping cough and diphtheria, were massively successful.[38] (See Appendix 1: Causes of Infant Death in Canada, for five year periods, 1921-50.) Valerie Minnett and Mary-Anne Poutanen have shown how children's active participation in efforts to eradicate disease-spreading houseflies in turn-of-the-century Montreal were pivotal to the success of anti-tuberculosis campaigns.[39] In many instances, as testimony in the proceeding chapters makes clear, the interventions of health professionals, educators, parents, and caregivers saved lives and/or immeasurably improved the quality of life for many children and their families. In 1900, 30.4 per cent of all deaths in Canada occurred among children younger than five years of age and the majority of these deaths were due to infectious diseases. By the late 1990s, that percentage was reduced to 1.4 per cent.[40] As the history explored here bears out, children's experiences with health and welfare interventions over the twentieth century were never simply reducible to "good" or "bad." Whether children benefited or not, placing their perspectives at the centre of analysis argues for a deeper appreciation of how shifting emphases in the discourse and enactment of good health made a difference on the body.

Although medical practitioners were not the only ones interested in children's health over the first half of the twentieth century, their professional discourse figures prominently as a historical source in this book. While both doctors and nurses were critical in the delivery of health services, doctors were particularly influential in inspiring and crafting public policy, guiding social agendas, and shaping the rhetoric and discourse surrounding it. The medical profession, Janice Hill argues, was "instrumental in naming, defining, and proposing strategies for the government of children."[41] Wendy Mitchinson has shown how the medical treatment of women at the hands of male doctors in Victorian Canada reflected attitudes towards gender and sexuality and, in turn, influenced women's place in the social order.[42] Mindful of Mitchinson's analysis, I argue that children were similarly influenced by the knowledge production of professional medical practitioners. Like the bodies of women, the bodies of children, according to doctors, were self-evidently deficient based on their differences in size and age, not simply from men, but from adults generally. For all their importance, however, doctors did not act in isolation. A range of medical practitioners; parents, siblings, and other relatives; educators; and community members contributed to and contested the embodiment of children as innocent, vulnerable, incompetent, and unpredictable – in sum, problematically different from adults. These forms of embodiment, in turn, had an impact on individual histories and familial decision making.

My focus is on the period between 1900 and 1940, with an emphasis on the interwar decades. It was during this time that a number of forces converged around the complex issue of child health: public health reform, efforts to control infant and maternal mortality, the rise of pediatrics as a medical specialty, the shift from control of contagious disease to the prevention of illness, and the entrenchment and evolution of "health" as a discrete curricular subject in public schools. Although the distinct character of Quebec often sets it apart from developments in Canada, Dominique Marshall has shown that the growth of the welfare state there was marked by similar intentions of protecting and enhancing strong, healthy children and families. The confluence of provincial compulsory schooling laws and federal family allowances marked the post-Second World War period as of particular importance in the development of welfare programs, but the Quebec state had a much longer history of promoting a protected childhood. Before the enactment of compulsory school law under Premier Adélard Godbout in 1943, children under sixteen years had to obtain a permit from the Quebec Department of Labour in order to work for a manufacturer or distributor. This enabled the state to better monitor young people leaving school to work. In larger cities such as Montreal, truant officers and school board enumerators enforced expectations of school attendance. In 1936, the Needy Mothers Assistance Fund was in place for poor mothers who could convince local authorities that they were among the "deserving poor."[43]

While professional and familial concern regarding the best way to preserve and cultivate children's health continued after the period under study, this book investigates the origins and early character of this confluence of forces. Although I do not offer a sustained comparative study of regional differences within the entire Canadian context, I am aware that place, including urban, rural, and regional, deeply mattered in the experience of youngsters and their families. Rather than a focus on formal social legislation regarding the structures of health and welfare reform (legislation that fell mainly under provincial jurisdiction), I highlight here the experience of the young with those responsible for ensuring and enhancing their health. This finer aperture should not, however, detract from my contention that the vision of healthy children promoted by professionals in schools and at home could and did transcend many boundaries. Finally, while young people in their teenaged years are occasionally considered, the focus of this book rests primarily with younger, elementary school-aged children.[44]

My analysis utilizes size and age as useful categories of analysis for historians of children and youth. In cultures influenced by white Anglo-Saxon and Anglo-Celtic traditions, children's embodied differences from adults are understood as natural, self-evident, and so taken for granted as not to merit comment or debate. In essence, few studies explicitly inquire after the changing meanings attached to children's size and age over time, or suggest how and why these meanings made (and make) children knowable in particular ways.[45]

Joan Scott's groundbreaking argument that gender, denoting the social organization of the relationship between the sexes, marked a useful category of analysis for historians, offers instructive parallels to my approach.[46] In this book, I explore how the embodied markers of size and age structured relationships between the generations and the differentials of power that sustained them.[47] While medical professionals were not the only adults who had a part in shaping children's experience with health, their powerful social place invested their views with potency. I argue that through their conceptualization, representation, and treatment of young, small bodies, medical and educational professionals contributed scientific legitimacy to the discursive construction of children as innocent, vulnerable, incompetent, and unpredictable. As David Michael Levin and George F. Solomon argue, the history of medicine is "inseparable from the fact that there have been, and still are, many different, often conflicting representations of the human body ... 'the body' which figures in medicine is always a discursive historical formation, a matter of selective representation; there is, in short, no totally 'natural' human body."[48] The construction of children's bodies, I argue, helped make unequal relations of power between children and adults sensible and "natural." Pathologies associated with infancy and childhood were in part guided by, and helped entrench, these ideological constructions and power differentials, along with racialized, classed, gendered, and able-bodied ideas about the "healthy child." From the perspective of youngsters and their families, this ideologically driven treatment resulted in a range of outcomes – not always positive – depending on one's social identity and location. Persuaded by Barrie Thorne's characterization of young age as a "form of embodied difference," I explore how, why, and with what consequences children's bodies were constructed in Canadian medical and educational discourse not simply as different, but as problematically and pathologically "not yet adult."[49]

A wide range of historical sources informs my analysis. The professional writing of doctors and nurses in medical journals and medical school textbooks, health curriculum textbooks recommended for use in Canadian public school classrooms, magazine and journal articles written by classroom teachers and other educational professionals, and a number of patient records from Toronto's HSC over the first four decades of the twentieth century comprise the textual sources utilized in the chapters that follow. I also make extensive use of oral history interviews. The oral histories included in this book were conducted with women and men from a range of backgrounds who grew up in various regions in Canada over the early years of the twentieth century up to the early 1960s (see Appendix 2: Participant Information).[50] Although the vast majority of subjects identified themselves as white Anglo-Celtic or white Anglo-Saxon, a number came from non-dominant groups, including those from First Nation communities, and immigrants from southern Europe and Asia. Also, given their longer life expectancy, interviews with women outnumber those with men. Those who grew up in rural and/or urban communities are both represented here, as are a range of class experiences, from impoverishment to affluence. While many grew up in families with a mother, father, and often siblings, some did not. Aunts and uncles, grandparents, or a lone parent, typically a mother, also raised some of the participants in this study.

I have acknowledged in my previous work, as have other scholars, that adult memories of growing up are not the same as historical evidence generated by youngsters in their childhood years.[51] George Morgan warns that "both oral testimony and the resultant written history are culturally encoded ... interviewees do not simply recite facts ... the process of remembering and speaking of the past is, like history writing, shaped by contemporary concerns and social processes (including collective/communal influences)."[52] In the absence of a rich repository of childhood testimony from the period, however, oral histories do invite different questions about the past, illuminating overlooked, ignored, and silenced perspectives. Privileging memories of growing up as key primary sources rather than marginalized anecdotes in historical interpretation positions the young as agents, however mediated, partial, and contingent, rather than passive objects of historical change over the twentieth century. Acknowledging the complex interaction between experts and the targets of their proscriptions, Ian Hacking reminds us that identities are not simply imposed "from above." There is, he acknowledges, a vector of labelling from above, from a community of experts who create a "reality" that some people make their own. Different from this is the vector of the autonomous behaviour of the person so labelled, which presses from below, creating a reality every expert must face.[53]

Focused primarily on articles in medical journals, including nursing journals, and medical textbooks, the first chapter of this book investigates how doctors and nurses characterized the young and their bodies, how they described their illnesses and injuries, what kinds of diagnoses and treatments were recommended, and what assumptions about their nature and capacity guided professional judgments. The representation of child bodies as "not yet adult" in medical literature was, I argue here, productive along two critical fronts: it supported the development of pediatrics as a separate medical specialty, and it positioned infancy and childhood as temporary pathologies, or illnesses, marked by embodied vulnerability, volatility, and danger. Assumptions associated with size and age combined with categories of gender, class, race, ethnicity, and ability to shape the experience of youngsters. As the following chapters will explore in more detail, children and their families benefited from, but were also challenged by, the consequences of medicine's tendency to pathologize the young and the small.

Memories of childhood form the focus of chapters 2 and 3. Chapter 2 explores the memories of Florence, Marc, Alice, and Theresa who grew up in the early years of the twentieth century, while chapter 3 explores the memories of Shirley, Lily, Jack, and Lina whose childhoods covered the late 1920s up to the end of the 1940s.[54] In these two chapters, childhood memories form the centre of the triangular interplay among youngsters, professional medicine, and what I call "domestic doctoring," or home care, most often provided by mothers, but also by fathers, grandparents, or siblings. These chapters are organized into two broad time periods that correspond generally with generational shifts, and shifts in approaches to children's health on the part of professionals.

The childhood memories of the eight adults highlighted in chapters 2 and 3 convey both shared and unique experiences with health care over the early to mid-twentieth century. The central role played by families is the most important common theme amongst the participants. Bouts of epidemic disease and chronic illness took on differing meanings within different families and shaped family routines and strategies for survival. Albeit in varying degrees, each participant recalled their parents or caregivers drawing on a mixture of folk and professional wisdom to treat pain and/or discomfort. Family members demonstrated understandable concern for their afflicted children, providing folk remedies and physical therapies. Mothers particularly, regardless of class affiliation, were remembered as skilled practitioners of various kinds of domestic doctoring. Unique aspects of the memories tend to bring sharply into relief the role of gender, race, and class in shaping how youngsters experienced various health challenges. Along with sexuality and ability, these markers of social identity are important throughout the book, but are particularly underscored in these two main chapters.

In conjunction with domestic doctoring and medical interventions, public education had a major impact on prevailing conceptions of "the healthy child." While school features prominently in the oral history chapters, it is front and centre in chapter 4. Here, I investigate the part that health education played in this process of fostering healthy children. The evolution of health curriculum remains largely unexplored in the Canadian context, despite the fact that it was added to the public school curriculum in the late 1800s. Often written in partnership with medical professionals, health textbooks conveyed hegemonic conceptions of good health, disease prevention, morals, and values. In health classes, students learned about their bodies, proper nutrition, the nature of disease-causing germs and bacteria, and the rules of public health and hygiene. They were measured, weighed, and inspected for dirt and lice, received vaccinations, eye examinations, and endured the extraction of teeth.

Health textbook curriculum, reflecting hegemonic social values, influenced how school children thought about and cared for their bodies. Christian tenets of self-control, cleanliness, and adherence to "rules" appropriate to the respectable classes were promoted in health curriculum early in the century. After the end of the First World War, and in the midst of considerable social change, new themes emerged. Changing scientific understandings of germ theory and disease prevention and new educational philosophies inspired health curriculum that aimed to persuade children to embrace healthy lives. Healthy living, in turn, was thought to act as a conduit to strong national identity and democratic citizenship, an important theme in the Second World War period. Social acceptability, the interests of the state, and so-called "good health" were manifest in children's physical health. The memories of women and men who attended public schools over roughly the first half of the twentieth century provide some sense of how youngsters responded to these shifting priorities. For reasons I explore in this chapter, some children folded health curriculum messages into their family life with relative ease. Others found themselves at odds with such messages.

Chapters 5 and 6 concentrate on two aspects of children's embodied experiences that emerged as important themes in the oral histories but that have received very little historical attention in the context of children's experiences in Canada: hospitalization and disability.[55] While mental disabilities are given some attention in chapter 6, the emphasis is on the experience of children with physical disabilities. Children requiring hospitalization and those with physical disabilities were similarly conceptualized over the twentieth century as "broken" and in need of "fixing." While treatment in hospital could bring great relief to sick and injured children, "fixing" those with disabilities was far less straightforward. Nevertheless, children with physical disabilities often spent much of their early years in hospitals seeking out and/or undergoing medical interventions aimed at improving their bodies. Over the period under study, medical professionals, parents, and children themselves, helped co-construct disability as a serious threat to health, normalcy, and well-being generally.

Hospitals were, and continue to be, important institutional sites for the protection and enhancement of children's health. They were never, however, the only place for such important preoccupations. Certainly as the oral histories demonstrate, domestic doctoring was far more likely the first response to illness or injury over the first half of the century. Nevertheless, hospitalization was an important event in the life of a child and, as adult memories testify, one that was often a formative life experience. In conjunction with published material and the oral histories of adults who spent time in hospital during their childhood, chapter 5 also makes use of archival sources at Toronto's HSC, one of Canada largest and oldest institutions devoted to children's health care. Patient records dating from the early 1900s to the 1940s provide a unique and revealing window on children's experiences and adult attitudes towards their afflictions and "abnormalities."

Like hospitalized children, children highlighted in chapter 6 who grew up with a physical disability had to navigate social forces, including mainstream medical knowledge, which characterized their bodies not simply as different, but as "abnormal" and unhealthy.[56] Unlike hospitalized children, and despite much effort to affect a "cure," children with physical differences often did not recover from their (socially undesirable) condition. Despite significant shifts in medical understanding of disability over the decades, and a clear desire to assist children with disabilities, doctors, nurses, teachers, and curriculum specialists tended to reinforce a eugenic-inspired pedagogy of failure regarding "abnormal" children well into the 1940s. This pedagogy of failure maintained that physical and behavioural difference was a serious threat to individual health, public health, and the nation-state. Surveillance, containment, and treatment represented the approach to disability that professionals advocated repeatedly over the century. Oral history testimony from adults who grew up with a physical disability, often caused by poliomyelitis, suggest that while medical professionals held considerable power, the values and capacities of individual families were also important. Parents were invested in helping their children overcome barriers and to this end, availed themselves of much that medical science had to offer. As the experiences in this book suggest, however, neither they nor their children did so unthinkingly. Given that they had their own set of complex motivations, needs, and desires, children with disabilities presented unique challenges to efforts aimed at reform.

Adult efforts to manage children's "temporariness" and children's responses to this management was foundational to the evolving nation-state at the end of the nineteenth and into the twentieth centuries. Social leaders in governmental, medical, and educational circles were preoccupied with the well-being of youngsters, particularly in the context of their status as "citizens-in-training." Children and their families complied with, and troubled, the desires of experts, variously supporting, interrupting, rejecting, and transmuting their attempts at embodied management. The incorporation of youthful perspectives makes clear that ideological constructions of children and childhood in this era of health reform were not simply natural, neutral, nor inevitable. They have a discernable and instructive history and were communicated, realized, challenged, and/or altered most immediately upon and through experiences involving the body. Our understanding of the era under study is sharpened when we ask how and why children experienced and responded to imperatives, both public and private, regarding health. This line of questioning reveals the key role that youngsters played in the racialized, classed, and gendered contestations that shaped how health was lived.

I

Doctored Bodies: Professional Medical Discourse and Children's Embodied Difference

Turn-of-the-twentieth-century attention to public health and the reduction of infant mortality put the spotlight on the health needs of children in unprecedented public ways. Interest in children as a special medical population grew from these concerted efforts and then expanded to include the rise of pediatrics, mass education campaigns dealing with sanitation and hygiene, and the promotion of disease prevention. Eager to bring the science of hygiene to rapidly growing cities, health officials promoted cleanliness, proper sanitation, and contagious disease control as a matter of public protection. Children were both the targets of, and eager participants in, campaigns to rid cities of contagious disease.[1] In this context, doctors, nurses, social welfare workers, and educators took advantage of professional journals, conferences, textbooks, magazines, and newspapers to promote their understanding of modern, scientific approaches to children's bodies and their health needs.

Wendy Mitchinson has shown how the medical treatment of women at the hands of predominantly male doctors in Victorian Canada reflected and solidified attitudes towards gender and sexuality and, in turn, influenced women's place in the social order.[2] Similarly, children as a specific population were soon enveloped within professional medicine's expansion and influence. Across the country, pediatrics as a recognized medical specialization spawned separate departments in medical schools, attracted practitioners, encouraged new treatment protocols and technologies, including the promotion of hospital births, fostered groundbreaking knowledge regarding infant nutrition, control of contagious diseases, and preventative medicine. A consequence of the rise of pediatrics, an example of medicine's "dividing practices" in Michel Foucault's phrase, was a child knowable through the specialized discourse of professional medical diagnosis, treatment, and care.[3] Whether it helped mitigate illness and suffering, or reinforced oppressive relations of power (or did both simultaneously), medical discourse regarding child patients influenced how adults understood the nature, needs, and capabilities of youngsters.

In this chapter I explore how conventional medical practitioners characterized the bodies of infants and children in their professional discourse over approximately the first four decades of the twentieth century. I am attentive to the ways doctors and nurses characterized the young, how they described their illnesses and injuries, what kinds of diagnoses and treatments were recommended, what assumptions about their nature and capacity guided professional judgments, and how this changed over time. The representation of child bodies as not yet adult in medical literature was a constant theme. I argue that this was productive along two critical fronts: it supported the development of pediatrics as a separate medical specialty, and it positioned infancy and childhood as temporary pathologies, marked by embodied vulnerability, volatility, and danger. Assumptions associated with size and age combined with categories of gender, class, race, ethnicity, and ability to shape the experience of youngsters. As proceeding chapters will explore in more detail, children and their families benefited from, but were also challenged by the attention of medical practitioners and their attempts to improve children's health.

FROM PROBLEM TO PREVENTION: PEDIATRICS, PUBLIC HEALTH, AND THE MOVE TO INTERVENTION

Historians of medicine have shown that home remedies for the succour of sick children developed and circulated in antiquity. Their application fell primarily to mothers and wet nurses in the domestic sphere.[4] In the West, the emergence of trained pediatric medical professionals began in earnest in the nineteenth century, at turns cooperating with and usurping parental and community control over children's treatment.[5] Even though they endured over the centuries, competing traditions of care, including European folk remedies, Indigenous practices, and traditional Chinese medicines, were often denigrated and dismissed as "backward," "quackery," and "superstition" by professionalized practitioners.[6] Despite pediatric medicine's rise in prominence, domestic doctoring did not disappear. It was, however, ideally to be directed and overseen by an increasingly powerful medical profession. As Pye Henry Chavasse's popular manual, *Advice to a Mother on the Management of Her Children and on the Treatment of the Moment of Some of Their More Pressing Illnesses and Accidents* (1880) suggested, "the care and management, and consequently the health and future well-doing [sic] of the child, principally devolve upon the mother, 'for it is the mother after all that has most to do with the making or marring of the man.'"[7] Despite the fact that mothers were acknowledged as supposedly "natural" nurses to their children, they were increasingly expected, as the twentieth century unfolded, to take direction from predominantly white and male medical specialists.[8] By the 1920s, for example, infant care in the context of hospitals supported by nurses and pediatricians was lauded as the ticket to successful and stress-free childrearing.

> Good nursing, together with regular feeding and the advent of the pediatrician renders remote the "walking of the floor all night with the crying baby." This is particularly true where the baby has gone through the regular routine of a first class hospital, so that the good technique observed can be carried out at home.[9]

Poor or abandoned children depended upon the philanthropic largesse of more fortunate others. Institutional solutions promised alternatives to neglect or worse. Annemarie Adams, David Theodore, and Judith Young point out that in many Western nations, including Canada, middle-class reformers, rather than medical professionals, initiated the development of children's hospitals and dedicated wards early in the Victorian period.[10] Beginning with the Montreal General Hospital's thirty-bed children's ward, opened in 1822, medical institutions entirely or partially devoted to children developed in major cities across the country over the turn of the twentieth century.[11] The development of institutional sites for the medical treatment of children invariably concentrated the interests and efforts of individual doctors inclined to focus on the young.

Beginning in the province of Quebec and spanning decades, medical faculties at universities around the country slowly developed dedicated pediatric training. In 1879, a clinical teaching course "for the care of the infant up to six months of age" was initiated at the medical faculty of Laval University in Quebec City, followed in 1894 by the establishment of the first chair of pediatrics in Canada. In 1895, Dr René Fortier, professor of pediatrics, took up the chair.[12] Even though the Canadian Society for the Study of Diseases of Children did not officially form until 1922, Dr A.D. Blackader, lecturer at McGill University in Montreal, joined the newly formed American Pediatric Society (APS) in 1888 and, by 1892, served as its president. He brought the meetings to Montreal in 1896 and in 1912 would be appointed the university's first professor of pediatrics. Dr Alan Brown, a pioneer of pediatric care at the Hospital for Sick Children (HSC), was appointed associate professor of pediatrics in the larger Department of Medicine at the University of Toronto in 1904. By 1935, pediatrics would finally be established as a separate department at the University of Toronto's Faculty of Medicine. Other faculties of medicine across the country slowly followed suit, developing courses, and then departments, of pediatrics.[13] As Howard Markel has shown, a similar pattern unfolded in the United States. There, "approximately five hundred physicians either practiced pediatrics exclusively or devoted 50 per cent or more of their professional efforts to caring for children" by the first decade of the twentieth century.[14]

As the twentieth century dawned, shifting attitudes towards acceptable standards of public health and rates of infant mortality bolstered pediatric specialization and professional attention to child health and welfare more generally.[15] Approximately one out of every five-to-seven babies died in the first year or two of life in Canada at the turn of the century.[16] The rates were even higher in Quebec, where one-in-three infants died before their third birthday. In 1900, the city of Montreal, for example, had a reputation as the "most unhealthy city in Canada," characterized by working-class families living in slums with extremely high rates of infant mortality. Tuberculosis, for example, claimed 135 out of every thousand deaths of youngsters between the ages of five and fourteen early in the century.[17] Infants with parents at the bottom of the socio-economic scale or who were Indigenous, tended to have higher rates of mortality.[18] Overall, the high rate of infant mortality was a state of affairs largely accepted as tragic, but not yet a matter of public concern. "What actually prevailed," Neil Sutherland has argued, "was a vague but generally unstated sense of inevitability and resignation."[19] By 1916, however, practitioners such as Dr Alan Brown signaled that such professional resignation was neither acceptable nor defensible. Addressing a nursing convention in Winnipeg, Manitoba in 1916, Brown noted critically

> how frequently one hears the assertion that delicate infants should not live; that efforts directed along this line are futile, and that hospitals erected for the saving of these delicate children are but mis-guided pieces of philanthropy, and in fact, some go so far as to state that it interferes with the law of natural selection which is the survival of the fittest.[20]

Brown advocated a different approach that positioned the work of professional practitioners as central and critical. Pediatric specialists would act as conduits, bringing public health concerns in line with special attention to the young and increased surveillance of home conditions.

Parental influence on the health of children was of constant concern to doctors and nurses. Poor, working-class, and racialized families – and mothers in particular – were most often represented in professional medical discourse as unable or unwilling to follow the rules of health, thus compromising new standards of child and infant care.[21] "Most of those who in infancy are regarded as physically unfit," Brown suggested, "were healthy at birth and merely the victims of a bad environment, improper feeding, and neglect, in short, conditions which it is quite possible to reverse."[22] Thus early in the new century, the provision of particular standards of health for Canadian children, as Cynthia Comacchio and Neil Sutherland have argued, was part of a broader set of state-sponsored social reform goals aimed at entrenching the values and standards of the white middle class.

Like their international counterparts in Britain and the United States, Canadian medical experts saw the convergence of unsanitary conditions in burgeoning cities, declining birth rates, increasing infant mortality, the death toll exacted by the First World War, and the arrival of large numbers of new immigrants as high prices to pay for modernity.[23] Troubled by the death toll exacted during the First World War, commentators in newspapers and the popular press called for increased attention to the general health of the nation, and children in particular. Writing in a Victoria, BC newspaper in 1919, an editorial writer summarized the cautious optimism and confidence that justified new health interventions:

> The new public conscience in matters of health demands that the indifference which permits such conditions must cease, that these uncorrected physical defects must be corrected, that there must exist no avoidable malnutrition among the children of this great Country. These young citizens must immediately be put into good physical shape and at the same time trained to take care of themselves, that they may go through life with a maximum of health and efficiency and joy in living.[24]

Infant and maternal welfare movements, dominated by white, Protestant, middle-class reformers and professionals, and backed by the public health research they provided, reconceptualized the high infant mortality rate as entirely unacceptable and in need of immediate improvement.[25] Many leading pediatric practitioners in North America, exemplified by the likes of American Emmett Holt and French Canadian Ernest Couture, joined the ranks of those who saw high rates of infant mortality as a matter of neglect and/or ignorance.[26] It was parental failure to accept and mimic new standards of healthy interaction with offspring that represented the greatest stumbling block to progress. Writing in the *Canadian Public Health Journal* in 1922, Holt, author of the influential and much reprinted *The Care and Feeding of Infants* (1894), *The Diseases of Infancy and Childcare* (1896), and co-founder of the American Pediatrics Society, implored doctors to win parental acceptance of the "principles of hygiene." Only then, Holt argued, would infant mortality, along with a host of other health issues, including venereal disease, hookworm, and tuberculosis, be brought under control. Doctors could do their part, Holt argued, but they had their work cut out for them. Underscoring the fact that health discourse reflects the social context in which it is embedded, Holt suggested that "some of these [bad habits] are racial," by which he meant emanating from non-Anglo-Celtic communities, "and have the sanctity of long usage but need to be altered to meet the changed conditions of modern life ... these rest on no other basis than prejudice, superstition, and there are no reasons for their continuance."[27]

The longstanding influence of eugenics – the cultural policing of the country's "genetic stock" – lent its support to a number of public health initiatives that institutionalized white, middle-class health priorities as the ultimate goal for families in Canada.[28] At the turn of the century, doctors looked to the health status of individual parents for clues to the inherited fate of the child. An 1897 medical school textbook used in Canada and penned by Henry Ashby and G.A. Wright suggested that

> an infant may come into the world fairly well developed and plump, from the presence of more or less stored-up fat, in spite of the weakly state of the mother's health, but it is almost certain sooner or later to exhibit tendencies to disease in the direction of the stock from whence it springs ... from its parents the foetus may receive the virus of syphilis ... it may receive an inheritance of tuberculosis or epilepsy, or a tendency to gout or rheumatism.[29]

Addressing the Alberta Medical Association in 1916, J.D. Dunn, medical inspector of Edmonton's public schools argued that protecting the future citizens of the country was the rightful responsibility of medical professionals. Parents could not always be trusted to do what was needed. Fears of "race suicide" lent support for increased surveillance and intervention into homes judged inadequate.

It is to be hoped that before many years have passed, we will have the satisfaction of seeing our ruling bodies give as much care and attention to the rising generation as they now give to the development of the best strains of livestock ... Should we allow the child to suffer and perhaps be handicapped for life through the ignorance or indifference of the parent? I do not think any of us would answer this question in the affirmative. We all know that this is the children's generation, and it is not very many years since the treatment of children received but very little attention. These children are the future parents and many of them would have a right to rise up and curse their parents as well as all others responsible for not doing their duty by them.[30]

By the 1930s, professionals understood that the battle against high rates of infant mortality would only be won by preventative measures in conjunction with the treatment of illnesses. Both options, however, required an increased level of medical intervention into the lives of Canadians. In his statistical portrait of child health in Canada for 1937, Ernest Couture, author of the widely distributed *The Canadian Mother and Child* and director of the Division of Child and Maternal Health, compared Canada's infant death rate to that of twelve other nations. Canada, with a rate of seventy-one deaths for every thousand live births, although a marked improvement from the past, still ranked ninth behind New Zealand (31), Australia (38), Sweden (46), the United States (54), the Union of South Africa (white) (57), England and Wales (58), Demark (66), and Ireland (except Northern Ireland) (73). Much work, cautioned Dr Couture, needed to be done. Citing a study by Winnipeg physician Dr T. McGinness on the autopsies of two hundred stillborn infants, causes of death were found to range from intracranial hemorrhage, to prematurity, to asphyxia, to congenital syphilis. "A proportion of lives," Couture maintained, "might have been saved through proper prenatal and intranatal care."[31] The prevention of illness or injury, Couture's comments make clear, was increasingly in line with professional emphasis on the considerable vulnerabilities associated with the young. It demanded a reorientation of the tasks of parenting and doctoring that stressed the anticipation and thus prevention of health problems. Nevertheless, the long-term decline in the infant mortality rate in Canada would have undoubtedly pleased and impressed Couture: between 1901 and 1997 the rate fell from 135 deaths per thousand to 5.5 deaths per thousand.[32] Rates for infant death caused by communicable diseases (including major killers such as measles, whooping cough, scarlet fever, diphtheria, and influenza) steadily declined between 1931 and 1945 from 743 to 449 per hundred thousand population.[33]

SIZE, AGE, AND PATHOLOGY IN PROFESSIONAL MEDICAL DISCOURSE

By the early decades of the twentieth century, as the writings of prominent doctors such as Alan Brown, Emmett Holt, and Ernest Couture suggest, professional interest in infants and children as medical populations with distinct and urgent health needs due in significant part to changing attitudes towards the prevention of infant death, was well-established. Doctors, encouraged to bring the infant care habits of uninformed or recalcitrant parents in line with standards dominated by mainstream science, were key architects of new standards of health surveillance that separated out youngsters for particular attention.

Medical textbooks and scientific journals provided reasons beyond the preservation of infant life for specialized attention to the young. The main rationale for the development of a pediatric specialization was the understanding that child and infant bodies were markedly different from adult bodies and that those differences could prove pathological. Merely being small and young, in other words, required medical attention. In his 1889 *Manual of Obstetrics, Gynaecology, and Paediatrics*, for example, Kenneth Fenwick focused specifically on the distinctions between younger and older bodies. It was the latter, however, that provided the standard measure of health and normalcy:

> While the infant may be regarded physically as the abstract of the man, possessing the same organs, the same processes of waste and repair, of growth and decay, still there are some important structural and functional differences between childhood and

adult life which modify and alter the diseases to which the young child is liable. Thus in childhood the tissues are softer, more vascular, and more succulent; the glandular, lymphatic, and capillary systems are extremely active; the skin and mucous membranes are softer, more delicate, and more sensitive; the brain is large, vascular, and almost fluid in consistency; there is excessive nervous excitability due to want of controlling power; and reflex sensitivity is excessively acute.[34]

The developmental distance between infants and children on one hand, and children and adults on the other marked the distance between embodied danger and healthy maturity. Focusing the attention of medical students on the risks of infant mortality, Henry Ashby and G.A. Wright warned at the turn of twentieth century that "the change from placental alimentation to the digestion of food in the infant's stomach is a time of peculiar danger, especially if artificial food is given and the mortality of infants is much greater during the first week of life than at any other period."[35] Other systemic liabilities posed equally serious challenges to infant viability. Despite considerable growth and change from the prenatal period, for example,

the mental faculties are in abeyance and the movements mostly involuntary or reflex. One consequence of the undeveloped condition of the higher or inhibitory centers is that the reflex centers are less under control than in later years, so that disorderly reflex movements in the form of convulsions are liable to take place on the slightest provocation.[36]

The representation of the small infant body as pathologically vulnerable to poor health, exemplified in Fenwick, Ashby, and Wright, influenced professional approaches over subsequent decades. Writing for the *Public Health Journal* in the mid-1920s, Dr George Smith remarked that

one should point out and emphasize the frailty of the material one is working with. Anatomically the infant lends itself to infection. The organs are small and almost fragile. The distance from the nose to the lung is very short. The physiological and mechanical resistance to oncoming infection is slight.[37]

In *Diseases of Childhood* (1926), Canadian Hector Charles Campbell warned, "at the moment of birth there is risk both of trauma and infection."[38] Young children, he argued, were born vulnerable to a triad of complications that vexed the doctor and parent alike throughout childhood: dietetic disturbances, infections, and severe emotional unrest.[39] "The metabolism of all children, just because they are children," he concluded, "is less stable than that of later life."[40] Should an infant also lack restful sleep, Campbell argued in a 1931 article in the *Canadian Medical Association Journal*, the culmination of physiological instability and emotional challenges could prove very difficult:

> But here, as so often happens in infancy, cause and effect are hard to separate, and we are confronted with a vicious circle of symptoms, each productive of the other. The infant, in the first months of life, functions almost solely as a suction apparatus ... Brought to the breast sleepless, crying, and excited, the child stammers in its attempt at suction ... Gulping, straining, and choking, it secures from the breast a minimum of milk and a maximum of air. The consequent distention of the stomach is painful.[41]

A happy, contented infant, Campbell's description suggests, depended on many interconnected, yet sometimes allusive conditions. The baby, represented in machine-like terms as "almost solely a suction apparatus," was unable to perform this key definitive function if deprived of restful sleep. The stakes for ensuring adequate amounts of infant sleep were high for parents, and for mothers in particular. It was at her breast, after all, that the baby would either find success or painful disappointment. Campbell's characterization of the infant was echoed in Alan Brown's influential manual, *The Normal Child: Its Care and Its Feeding* (1923). As Norah Lewis has argued, Brown

> reflected the *Tabula Rasa* point of view accepted by many advisors of the early 1920s when he described newborns as not being

directly aware of anything, having little more intelligence than a vegetable, unable to distinguish light and darkness, but equipped with a slight sense of smell and a well-developed sense of taste.[42]

Should children require the attention of a physician, other significant challenges attended their medical treatment. Kenneth Fenwick warned medical students in great detail about the nearly insurmountable difficulties that attended the accurate medical diagnosis of ailments in babies and children. The crux of the difficulties had to do with the inherent inadequacies of the young. They could not, doctors warned, communicate effectively with adults. It was up to well-trained and patient medical professionals to unravel their diagnostic mysteries:

> While the diagnosis is often a difficult task in the adult, it is still much more so in the infant where our only guide is an objective examination ... So great are these difficulties in the clinical examination of children that unless you have been prepared by some preliminary study you will find it a most uncertain and disheartening task to unravel the history and nature of any case that may come to you. The task is one which requires patience, good nature, and tact, for the helpless silence of the infant, the incorrect answers of the older child, the fright, agitation, or anger produced by your examination, or even mere presence, render it difficult to detect the real aberration of function. And lastly, the difficulty of obtaining reliable information from the mother or nurse all concur to make your examination of children, with a view to find the seat of disease, a most difficult and perplexing one.[43]

The attitudes and assumptions guiding Fenwick's warnings are revealing. He is careful to underscore the necessity of specialized pediatric training for those practitioners who care for the young. Without it, he suggests, efforts to accurately diagnose childhood afflictions are compromised. Presented principally as medical problems, infants and children confounded and challenged the doctor's best efforts and reacted unpredictably to examination. Seemingly afflicted with similar shortcomings, mothers and nurses were thought to be rather poor mediators.

Echoing Fenwick's early pronouncements on the challenges of pediatric diagnosis, Alan Brown and Fred Tisdall advised doctors in *Common Procedures in the Practice of Paediatrics*, first published in 1929, that "the physical examination of infants and children presents many problems quite distinct from those encountered in the examination of adults."[44] They seemed more confident, however, that the specialized training afforded the pediatrician could overcome patient inadequacies. A successful diagnosis could be made, regardless of whether or not the patient was co-operative. Young patients, they advised, needed thorough "inspection" from head to toe. Judging the child's cry – its intensity and tenor – was a valuable tool for diagnosis:

Much information can be obtained by observing the child while the mother is being questioned. If the patient is crying vigorously or taking an interest in its surroundings you know at once that it is not acutely ill. In regard to the character of the cry, with a little practice it is possible to determine whether it is due to the patient being hungry or in pain or whether it is merely the result of fright or temper.[45]

That neither mothers nor children could describe the causes of discomfort or illness satisfactorily enough for practitioners did not preclude successful diagnosis for modern professionals. Brown and Tisdall insinuated that in fact the perspective of the sick child or their parent was quite incidental to successful medical practice. Commenting on the under-diagnosis of peptic ulcers in children in the 1940s, Dr O.M. Moore from the Department of Pediatrics at Vancouver General Hospital made clear that children, by their very nature, could not only be difficult to decipher, they were also not to be trusted. Some of the blame for this rested with medical professionals, such as roentgenologists – radiologists – who were "unlikely to have gastrointestinal series done in children" due to their "natural conservatism." Other aspects of the problem, however, reflected deeply held beliefs about the nature of children themselves: children were "renowned for dietary imprudence"; they were unable to "accurately describe symptoms of discomfort"; and were "inaccurate in describing and localizing pain," and "particularly susceptible to suggestion" – "they should be asked no 'leading' questions unless it is unavoidable."[46] Not only did small size render the young inherently susceptible to illness and disease, qualities of character associated with their age challenged professionals' ability to safeguard their health and well-being.

By the end of the 1930s, youngsters emerged from the professional discourse of pediatric specialists as a population whose embodied vulnerabilities and liabilities had for too long been misunderstood and underestimated. In their repudiation of these kinds of outdated attitudes, and undoubtedly in defense of their own work, doctors encouraged adults – parents and practitioners in particular – to be ever mindful of, and to take responsibility for, the dangers to health that being young and small presented. Dr Alan Brown lambasted insensitive (and ignorant) adults, lay and professional alike, who endangered vulnerable babies:

> How common is the experience that fathers, grandmothers, aunts, children, etc., gather round to "gloat" over the new addition to the family and during the process distribute, or better "spew," their germs from their noses and throats (they are usually some of them suffering from some type of nose or throat infection) directly on to the new-born infant, who has not been sufficiently long in its new environment to develop any immunity, and the next thing we hear is that the "poor baby died of pneumonia."[47]

Emphasizing the vulnerabilities of infants, Brown hoped to shame his readers into engaging more seriously and mindfully with the prevention of infection and disease. Advertisers took great advantage of such calls for new standards of hygiene, directly linking commercial products such as Kleenex, Vicks VapoRub, and Zam-Buk ointment with medical efforts to stop, or at least lessen, the spread of colds and influenza:

> Stop risking your children's health! Adopt the protection doctors and nurses recommend – use Kleenex during a cold ... It holds

germs. They can't get away, can't spread your cold ... you use a fresh, gentle Kleenex Tissue each time. Destroy it, and destroy germs with it![48]

The same preventative orientation was advocated in the case of older children. Dr Lloyd P. MacHaffie, Ottawa's school medical officer, for example, was particularly invested in ensuring that by the time children entered school, they were largely free of congenital health problems. Illnesses left untreated or simply dismissed as part of growing up, MacHaffie warned, entirely underestimated the vulnerability and volatility of children's bodies. In a 1936 article entitled, "Pitfalls and Tragedies of the Pre-School Child," MacHaffie made it very clear that such outdated attitudes came with a very high cost:

While the child was outgrowing diseased tonsils, his heart was being damaged beyond repair; that while outgrowing malnutrition, his body would be a fertile receptive soil for germs of all types; that while outgrowing ear-ache and bealing ears, he would gradually grow into permanent deafness; that while outgrowing a squint, he was growing blind; and that while outgrowing pains – which usually are rheumatism – he would develop heart disease; and so on *ad infinitum* with the pathetic story.[49]

Over the course of the twentieth century, the preventative orientation to youth health was promoted as paramount. In the case of infants and children, prevention was imbued with a moral duty to protect those represented as the most vulnerable and the most susceptible to health problems. Writing in the CMAJ in 1943, for example, Dr Nelles Silverthorne reported that all of the 368 children diagnosed with tubercular meningitis between 1940 and 1943 had died. "The only method for control of this disease is its prevention," Silverthorne wrote. "Much has been done in this respect in the last few years in the control of active cases, in the pasteurization of milk, and in the education of the public to the danger to children of contact with tuberculosis."[50]

Other practitioners took a sometimes less optimistic tact. In an article in *The Canadian Nurse* published at the end of the 1940s and entitled, "Rheumatic Fever: The Scourge of Childhood," Olive B. Warren, a student nurse at Sarnia General Hospital, echoed the warnings to parents that had characterized the writings of other professionals decades earlier. Warren sharply warned that in order to protect the young from serious health complications, parents needed to take their complaints seriously: "These weak harbingers of a serious condition are the so-called 'growing pains' which are dismissed lightly by many parents as a normal phase of childhood."[51] Like other health professionals, Warren advocated a reconceptualization of children as far more pathological and prone to problems than previously thought or that many parents seemed to accept.

CONTEXTUALIZING THE PATHOLOGY OF SMALL, YOUNG BODIES

Attitudes towards gender, race, class, and ability added complex layers of meaning to understandings of representations of youthful embodied pathologies. While medical professionals identified clear pathologies associated simply with youth and size, boys and girls were believed to suffer specific challenges based on gendered constraints. The tyranny of fashionable styles, for example, was singled out by turn-of-the-century medical and educational professionals as particularly detrimental for girls. Some cautions sprang from newly understood dangers. Pye Henry Chavasse brought to the attention of parents the deadly consequences of green-dyed dresses for girls. "It is injurious," Chavasse warned, "to wear a green dress, if the colour has been imparted to it by means of Scheele's green, which is arsenite [sic] of copper – a deadly poison ... I have known the arsenic to fly off from a green dress in the form of powder, and to produce, in consequence, ill-health."[52] A manual aimed at older students similarly drew attention to the negative consequences of the common turn-of-the-century practice of corseting and using garter belts:

> Tight-lacing, as practiced too frequently by girls, until the waist looks like an hour-glass, and as easy to snap as a pipe-stem, results in dangerous compression of all the vital organs, and must, if preserved in, end in disease and deformity. Tightness of

any article of dress is particularly to be guarded against in children, in whom the bones are soft and easily bent out of their proper shape. Garters are apt to induce varicose veins, and also spoil the shape of the leg.[53]

While boys were not completely exempt from such gendered admonitions in terms of fashion, they tended to be less serious. In the same manual, for example, boys were reminded "in male attire, the belting of the trousers is also injurious. Head covering such as tight fitting silk or beaver hats, made of substances which are non-conductors of heat, retain the heated air in contact with the head, and by compression frequently give rise to headaches."[54]

Early twentieth century health textbooks approved for use in Canadian schools promoted attitudes and activities that improved health while observing gendered expectations.[55] While authors championed the idea that physical exercise was important for the maintenance of good health, they differentiated types of exercise and levels of exertion were assigned to boys and girls, particularly as they got older. "Girls should play and romp with the same freedom that boys do," wrote Dr William Krohn in a 1907 elementary grade health primer. "Health is as necessary to a girl as it is to a boy."[56] Dr Charles Stowell, the provincial secretary of health for the province of British Columbia similarly declared in a 1909 health text that a new era of health "emancipation" had dawned for women. "Not many decades ago the beautiful woman was supposed to have pale cheeks and a languid manner and to lead an indoor life," Stowell wrote, "but this anemic style of beauty has been supplanted by the rosy-cheeked athletic girl who spends as much time as possible in the open air."[57] Whereas boys were encouraged to engage in rough and tumble team sports, girls were to seek out more modest and controlled physical pursuits.[58]

The promotion of regular outdoor exercise, balanced diets, cleanliness, and plenty of sleep in childhood was cast as an investment in the future. Healthy girls and healthy boys grew into strong wives and mothers, and capable, robust husbands and fathers. By the end of the First World War, for example, public health officials took full advantage of school health programming to teach proper techniques of modern mothering. Speaking to fellow nurses at the Canadian Nursing Association (CNA) conference in Winnipeg in 1916, Nora Moore argued:

> If better conditions are to exist in our schools five, ten years hence, we must begin to create those conditions now. This was one of the motives prompting the institution this year of "Little Mothers' Classes," a branch of our work that has already had gratifying results. In 19 schools our nurses are conducting these classes in rooms equipped with bath tub, hospital cot, weighing machines, etc. Little girls of ten and over gather about and receive practical instruction in every step of the process of washing and dressing an infant, first using large celluloid dolls until showing themselves careful and sufficiently capable to have a "real live baby" entrusted to them.[59]

Whereas both boys and girls were susceptible to various diseases, gendered differences were marshalled to account for variations in rates and experiences. Dr J. Wyllie reported in the *Canadian Public Health Journal* in 1933, for example, that "tuberculosis is more fatal for girls than for boys in this age period [five to fourteen years] but inspite of the high female tuberculosis rate the general male mortality rate is slightly higher than the general female rate. This is accounted for by the greater number of accidental deaths among boys, who are more daring and reckless than girls."[60] In a survey of the food consumption of a number of low-income families in Toronto in the early 1940s, gendered attitudes and behaviours played a major role in shaping the nutritional intake of all family members. The researchers discovered that

> except for vitamin B1, the diets of the younger children and of the teen-age boys were adequate. The calcium intake of the teen-age girls was low. The calcium requirement is greater in the teens than in the children under twelve because of the rate of skeletal growth. The milk consumption of the teen-age girls was low. The reason for this was easy to find; the girls wanted to be thin and they erroneously thought that milk was fattening.[61]

The desire for girls to adhere to conventional standards of beauty was thoroughly intertwined with broader issues of health. Linkages between them, however erroneous, were made by adults and by girls themselves. As Helen Boyd recalled,

> when it came time for my younger sister to be vaccinated, there was a fad at the school to have girls vaccinated on their thighs to avoid having the scar on the arm. I put on a campaign for this, pointing out how perfectly dreadful it was to have the effect of a beautiful ball gown spoiled by an ugly scar. Father thought the situation was exactly the opposite: "When I go to a ball I don't look at a women's dress, or even her ankles: I just look to see that she has a good healthy vaccination on her arm."[62]

Despite her father's attempts to reassure Helen that good health eventually led to beauty, other adults argued that in the case of girls, the two went hand-in-hand. Beautiful girls were healthy girls. In a 1932 *Chatelaine* magazine article entitled, "Beauty," author Annabelle Lee told readers that

> good looks are so intrinsically bound up with health. If we develop sound, strong bodies, beauty will follow of its own accord, and there will be only a little "finishing" to do. Babies nowadays have far more opportunity to grow into beautiful women than their grandmothers, or even their mothers had. A widespread knowledge of the essential elements of diet and hygiene is responsible for all the radiant, bonny babies one sees. There is every reason why they should be beautiful in maturity.[63]

Clearly in the case of girls, "sound, strong bodies" and adherence to the "essential elements of diet and hygiene" was rewarded with the promised added bonus of physical beauty. In this way, links among "normal" bodies, good health, beauty, and social value were insinuated.

While gender played a central role in shaping how medical professionals represented healthy children and healthy bodies, social class was also critical. Children in poor or working-class families, for example, were cast as simultaneously vulnerable to the poor choices of their parents and potentially dangerous to the health of surrounding communities. Nurse Nora Moore reported to the 1916 Winnipeg CNA,

> It has been a frequent experience with us to find a really serious disease, e.g. scarlet fever, by following up what was reported to us as a rash, especially in cases where families are poor, children neglected, probably both parents away all day working, and only by a visit from the nurse during the day has the disease been discovered and the children quarantined.[64]

As the work of Tamara Myers has shown, parents, for the most part from the "lower" classes, judged neglectful of their children or in any way contributing to their juvenile delinquency (however broadly defined), could be subject to juvenile court discipline.[65] In this way, professionals could draw on considerable resources to enforce their will. "Occasionally," as Nora Moore suggested, "things do not go so smoothly between nurse and parent, and after persistent refusal to have his child treated, if the nurse deems the child in danger, the father is summoned to the Juvenile Court, where law comes to the aid of the school nurse."[66] Professional practitioners tended to conceptualize these "other bodies" as not simply in need of good advice, but of significant discipline and occasional punishment.

The children of the immigrant working classes were particularly imperiled by their supposed embodied shortcomings. A potent example is offered in "In the Children's Ward," a feature story told from the perspective of Nurse B.E.A. Philmot, in *The Canadian Nurse* in April of 1909. In her account of the various children and families encountered on the ward, intertwined issues of ethnicity, class, and gender come to the forefront. Readers learn of the fate of Dennis, a three-year-old boy of working-class Irish descent early in the nurse's observations. According to Philmot,

> we undressed him by main force and put him in the tub. He evidently, to judge by his struggles, thought we were going to drown him. Probably he had never seen so much water collected in one

place before. Also he dreaded to part with that outer covering of dirt; it had been his own for so long it was well-nigh impossible to take it from him.[67]

Although Dennis eventually "learns" to be a proper patient, he cannot simply wash away his ethnic and class identity. Drawing on entrenched stereotypes surrounding acceptable masculinity and Irish-Canadian boys, the author notes that he will likely become "a prizefighter one day for he had just the figure for it!"[68]

Challenges to the provision of good health posed by those outside the boundaries of the white middle class were mitigated by efforts to change uncooperative behaviours, habits, and priorities. Advocating that parents take advantage of medical expertise *before* their child became sick, however, was not a straightforward reorientation of childrearing habits. Prevention, and the concomitant conceptualization of children as inherently prone to sickness, was shot through with constraints associated with class, race, ethnicity, and gender. Reporting to the Pediatric Section of the Canadian Medical Association in June of 1924, Dr A.P. Hart from Toronto spoke regretfully of the "difficulty in establishing a baby clinic amongst the foreign element of the population who did not appreciate a 'well-baby' clinic but rather waited until the infant was ill before seeking assistance."[69] Disregarding the limits of family budgets, Dr Grant Fleming, who promoted the value of regular visits to the family doctor, suggested in a 1929 article that individual responsibility for one's health was the order of the day. His promotion of "personal hygiene" traded firmly on a fundamental assumption that most people were economically placed to take advantage of "modern inventions" that were believed to enhance health:

> Individual health depends essentially upon the individual's practice of what we call "personal hygiene." Even in our age of organization, we expect that we must consider our bath, our bedtime, and our open bedroom window as personal responsibilities. Modern inventions have given us conveniences that greatly assist and make reasonably easy the practice of personal hygiene.[70]

Indoor plumbing with running water, separate bedrooms with windows, new household gadgets, sound diets, and choices regarding quality of sleep were assumed to be within reach of most, if not all, Canadians.

Children were expected to learn these principles of "personal hygiene" early and to eventually come to weave them into their daily routines. Health education in schools was cited as a particularly significant force in this regard. In an article reprinted in the *Canadian Public Health Journal* in 1922, Emmett Holt wrote,

> When a child has learned in school that to get up to his normal weight or to gain weight he must go to bed at eight o'clock and not play in the street till ten or eleven, that he must drink milk, not tea and coffee; eat regular meals and not fill his stomach with trash between meals; must eat a variety of food cereals, green vegetables, fruit, etc. ... does anyone for one moment believe that such habits formed in childhood during school life will not make a lasting impression upon the life of the individual?[71]

Like Fleming, Holt's optimism traded on the understanding that good health was simply a matter of learning positive health habits. His conviction, however, accentuated middle-class sensibilities. Families with the means to provide not only close supervision of their children but also a variety of foods equated to healthy families. Those who could not provide these things required significant reformation.

Assumptions about the health of First Nation peoples, including the belief that they were incapable of looking after their own health, underlined the role that race played in shaping attitudes towards the pathology of childhood. Indeed, many white medical professionals regarded First Nation peoples as actively disregarding or sabotaging their well-being. In a 1914 report to the Department of Indian Affairs regarding the conditions at Fisher River, Manitoba, for example, the agent made it quite clear that First Nation habits hindered development: "Taken as a whole the health is good but could be improved, and the ravages of consumption greatly lessened, if the

Indians could be induced to adopt common sanitary precautions and keep better ventilation in their houses during the winter months."[72] By the late 1920s, Indian agents and medical personnel targeted First Nation parents, particularly mothers, in an effort to teach them "the art of living." Reforming First Nation habits of parenting, it was hoped, would lower rates of infant mortality.[73]

Demands on First Nation peoples to improve health habits by abandoning traditional practices coexisted with their recurring neglect by white professional practitioners. Even as more and more people were moved to overcrowded and underserviced reserves, they disproportionately received the disadvantages, not the benefits, of professional attention. "There was no doctor at the Indian villages of Klemtu and Kitamaat, and these places were not receiving much in the way of medical attention," reported Florence Moffatt, a nurse at the R.W. Large Memorial Hospital on Campbell Island in British Columbia in the 1940s. When Moffatt visited these neglected villages, she struggled, often unsuccessfully, to help keep her patients alive: "I treated more than forty people with penicillin and mild sedatives. One young girl had a severe ear infection following a mastoid operation. I had taken her to the hospital, but the infection had been too severe and too longstanding, and she died shortly afterward."[74]

The increasing importance of nutritional science in the interwar period and assumptions about the superiority of Anglo-Celtic dietary habits made First Nation populations attractive targets for medical experiments. Writing about her nursing experiences in the Arctic over the 1930s and 1940s, Margery Hind reported on a study of the "effects of white man's food upon Eskimo children" undertaken by the white Toronto-based nurse stationed there. Each morning the children "received a bowl of porridge, half a pint of rich milk, a pilot biscuit, a vitamin pill, and a spoonful of cod liver oil ... these children are weighed regularly, and a special note is made of their ailments."[75] In a large study of the nutritional status of the First Nations of James Bay published in the prestigious *Canadian Medical Association Journal* in 1948, the authors suggested that

> many characteristics, such as shiftlessness, indolence, improvidence, and inertia, so long regarded as inherent or hereditary

traits in the Indian race, may at the root be really the manifestation of malnutrition. This is of concern not only to the Indian but to the white population, as any attempt to eradicate tuberculosis in Canada must include the institution of preventative measures for everyone. In addition, from the economic standpoint a group of people in poor health tends to be a liability rather than an asset to the nation.[76]

Medical studies of First Nation peoples' reactions to changes in diet appeared to unfold in tandem with their virtual neglect by professional medical practitioners in other contexts, such as the residential schools.[77] In a most ironically tragic twist, it was in the residential schools, institutions run by whites, where inadequate food was a common hardship endured by First Nation children.[78]

CONCLUSIONS

Over the first four decades of the twentieth century, medical professionals encouraged Canadians to take more seriously their children's health along a number of related fronts. First, by way of confronting rates of infant mortality, professionals encouraged fellow practitioners and parents alike to abandon old ways of thinking that took infant vulnerability to sickness and death entirely for granted. Professionals did so not by suggesting that infants were more resilient than given credit for, but by demonstrating that diagnosis and treatment of child and infant ailments had significantly progressed. Second, parents in particular were encouraged to reconceptualize their children as vulnerable to multiple health threats that could be caught early or even prevented with proper attention. Professional medical practitioners cast these new responsibilities for parents as particularly vexing given long-standing tendencies to view infancy and childhood as times of embodied vulnerability for which there was little remedy, save growing up. The aim was to present preventative health care and attention as a new orientation to the natural embodied needs of youngsters.

In their professional discussions, doctors and nurses represented infants and children as a challenging and critical medical demographic.

By virtue of size and age, young and small bodies were prone to disease and infection. They were volatile and unpredictable. In essence, they were not yet adult bodies and thus not yet, the reasoning went, stable, healthy, and normal. Even in the case of older children, diagnosis and treatment of illness constituted processes fraught with complications. Children themselves, according to the medical professionals charged with their care, did not reveal their embodied secrets easily nor accurately. Practitioners encouraged one another to develop the necessary diagnostic and treatment skills to treat the young with either very little or highly suspect input from patients themselves.

Important markers of social identity, including race, class, gender, and ethnicity, brought more finely calibrated meaning to the pathology associated with childhood. The definition of "good health" offered by medical professionals reflected their own privilege as leading members of the white middle class. Based on their distance from this ideal, infants and children racialized as non-white and/or from poor, working-class, or immigrant backgrounds were assumed to suffer additional health challenges. In the following chapters I concentrate more fully on the perspectives of youngsters from a variety of backgrounds as they learned to be healthy, endured illness and injury, and encountered medical practitioners. These perspectives complicate and temper medical professionals' tendency to render childhood a pathological condition. In some cases, and despite the best of intentions, adult interventions caused and/or exacerbated threats to health and well-being that confronted young people and their families.

2

Florence, Marc, Alice, and Theresa: Healthy Bodies and Domestic Doctoring, 1910s to the 1920s

As medical professionals worked to establish pediatric medicine as a legitimate specialization over the early decades of the twentieth century, children and their families encountered many health challenges. Multi-pronged responses to high rates of infant mortality, disease, and infection in the early twentieth century reflected new expectations for children's health and welfare, and supported a growing network of professionals dedicated to the task. Public health officials, doctors, nurses, social workers, well-baby clinic staff, school administrators, teachers, and others interacted directly and indirectly with families to improve health. As Cynthia Comacchio has argued, "child nurture and family health became state interests" in Canada over the early decades of the new century.[1] In this context, infancy and childhood emerged from professional medical discourse as life stages fraught with both health challenges and opportunities for intervention and improvement.

In this chapter and the next, I turn to the memories of adults who experienced both good and bad health in their childhood. Professional practitioners, traditional healers, family members, and neighbours worked hard to alleviate the suffering of children but their assumptions about children's nature, as the oral histories reveal, could also worsen a child's condition or otherwise compromise their sense of well-being. Attitudes towards race, class, gender, and "normalcy" also shaped this process in definitive ways. Despite these formidable forces, children themselves, as well as their families, took an active role in the decision-making process surrounding health and medical treatment. They did not simply wait on direction from professionals, even though professionals had considerable influence in their lives. As the oral histories explored here make clear, children variously endured, contemplated, and weighed the advice of doctors and nurses, parents, neighbours, and folk healers in relation to their own desires, hopes, and fears. The achievement and promotion of good health was important, but it was only one strand in the complex fabric of family life.

Each of the children profiled in this chapter were born in the midst of the First World War, although none spoke of its direct impact on family life. Florence, Marc, Alice, and Theresa were very young at the time of the war's outbreak and were preoccupied with other, more immediate events in their lives. In particular, the 1918 influenza pandemic, known as the Spanish flu, had a lasting impact on the life of Marc. Nevertheless, the war spurred on new protocols in public health, sanitation, and medical knowledge that contextualized children's experiences with health and welfare in Canada in this period.[2] Children's efforts to live with, and through, sickness and injury, always in relation to their own needs and capacities and those of their family, was a fundamental part of growing up in the new century.

FLORENCE

Florence Drake was born in Vancouver, British Columbia in 1908. Her father worked as a carpenter at Woodward's Department Store in the downtown core and her mother was a full-time homemaker. She was raised in a modest two-bedroom bungalow, comfortably ensconced in the then largely working-class neighbourhood of Grandview-Woodlands.[3] In 1910, when Florence was two years old, she contracted poliomyelitis. That year marked an outbreak of many cases of the disease around the country. As Christopher Rutty has documented, poliomyelitis tended to strike "the vigorous and healthy who lived in comfortable middle-class homes" which confounded public health officials "experienced with the dominant 'dirt and disease' model of infectious diseases."[4] Children would have to wait nearly a half-century before a safe and effective polio vaccine would be developed.[5]

The day that Florence became ill had begun with a trip to English Bay with her mother and siblings. The children had played on the beach all day and returned home, exhausted but happy. The next morning, Florence's mother was horrified to hear her young daughter screaming in pain, unable to stand. A frantic call to their doctor provided little comfort. The doctor reported that his son was experiencing similar symptoms. "He didn't know what was wrong, so he didn't come to the house or anything," Florence reported. "He said he didn't know what to do because it was all new to him, and he didn't know what it was."[6]

The majority of Florence's early childhood memories revolve around the numerous strategies adopted by her parents and medical professionals to mitigate polio's effects, particularly damage to her leg muscles. She remembers a woman coming to her house to treat her with electrotherapy when she was around four years old:

> She used to come on the street car, and she had a black box with her, and it was full of wires and I was scared to death of it. I hated it, and I used to run and hide when she came. And she would wind these wires all around my leg and then she would plug it in – into the electricity. And it was all pins and needles and everything all up and down my leg.[7]

Electrotherapy was developed late in the nineteenth century by Guilliaume Duchenne, a French neurologist, as a means of stimulating contractions of atrophied muscles. By the turn of the twentieth century, both legitimate and illegitimate practitioners used electrotherapy.[8] Florence could not remember whether the woman with the black box was a nurse or a lay practitioner. In either case, her parents likely paid for their daughter's treatment. In an era before the development of publicly funded health care and private medical insurance, affordable treatments were attractive if not always effective.[9] When the electrotherapy failed to stimulate her leg muscles, Florence, like many other polio survivors, was fitted with irons. Irons were braces that fit around the foot, inside the shoe, and extended up the side of her leg to her knee where it was fastened. She wore this brace for a number of years.

In 1919, at the age of eleven, Florence's parents took her to Vancouver General Hospital for a series of operations that would take place over the next two years. One doctor, Florence recalled, promised that he could help her gain back some of her physical mobility. "Well," she recalled her father saying to the doctor, "you go ahead because she has never had anything done for any of it ... I will just leave it in your hands and you do what you think you can do for her."[10] The trust that Florence's father displayed was a significant source of power and prestige for doctors and reflected the success of the profession's efforts in these years to establish its authority. As another respondent remembered, "You didn't argue with doctors in those days. And my parents really thought they were gods. Whatever doctors said, that was it."[11]

Despite this reputation, professional treatment, like lay treatment, did not guarantee results. Florence experienced this disappointment first-hand. The operations on her feet, for example, were only partially successful and left behind scars that ran from her toes around the front of her foot to her ankles. When the doctor proposed more operations to correct "weak knees," Florence balked. "I would have to lay on my back for one year while he put weights attached to my leg at the bottom of my bed ... this I refused," she said. In this instance, Florence was able to exercise her own "knee-high agency" regarding a major medical decision.[12] She had already missed two years of school by this point and would eventually end her schooling when she reached the eighth grade. Florence did not recall her parents disagreeing with her refusal; it is possible, given the expense, lack of expected results, and school disruptions, that they agreed with her. Noteworthy, nonetheless, particularly in the context of the ascendency of the power of pediatric professionals during the early decades of the century, was Florence's clear sense of her own power to refuse this particular intervention.

During her stay in the hospital, Florence saw her parents only once a week. They did not live close by, she recalled, and it was understood that they had to juggle competing demands of breadwinning and looking after her other siblings. Until well into the second half of the twentieth century, hospitalized children routinely spent long periods of time in care without educational or recreational programming to help ease familial separation, boredom, or fear.[13] An analysis of pediatric admissions to Kingston General Hospital in the province of Ontario between 1899 and 1909 suggests, however, that parents, particularly mothers, developed strategies to provide support. When children were admitted to Kingston General as pediatric cases, mothers were also often admitted and shared a room with their children for the duration of their stay. This practice became so common that a directive was issued by the government of Ontario in July of 1905 decrying it as a misuse of hospital beds. Thereafter, records of such admissions in the case of Kingston General dwindled and eventually ceased.[14]

Although Florence remembered her hospitalization as a time of great loneliness, she was proactive in her attempts to cope. Putting herself to work was one such strategy. "I was in a wheelchair," she remembered, "and of course it had the feet straight out and I used to put bedpans and napkins and stuff on my legs, and drop one off on each bed ... I would help the nurses and it was something for me to do."[15] Spending time on the hospital's glassed-in veranda also enabled her to meet other patients and befriend staff members. "I would see the ambulance coming, you know?" she recalled, "and I got to know the ambulance drivers."[16]

As Florence entered her teenaged years, the pressure to conform to gendered expectations around fashion and bodily appearance mounted. Although her uneven gait did not compromise her health, it was socially difficult given attitudes towards disability and the disabled as "abnormal."[17] When she had outgrown her leg braces, she took advantage of orthotic shoes available at Pierre Paris's shoe store on Hastings Street in Vancouver:

> He made me a pair of shoes and he built one boot a way up with cork. It was quite light in weight, but it was sure ugly looking. You see this is the hard part too when you are a teenager and everybody was dancing, and they wore – at that time they wore French heels like pumps? Black patent leather pumps? I couldn't wear anything like that. All I could wear was an old Oxford. So that limited your kind of dress. If you are going to wear Oxfords, you've got to have a suit or a skirt, and I could never wear what I wanted.[18]

Florence longed to be a full participant in the culture of her teenaged peers but this depended upon a non-disabled body. She was fully aware that she existed on the edges of acceptability and regretted being left out.

Coping with the effects of polio and its treatment preoccupied much of Florence's memories of growing up, but they were not the only health challenges she recalled. Around the age of five she was diagnosed with diphtheria, a contagious bacterial infection of the upper respiratory tract. The family was unceremoniously quarantined after the infection was diagnosed. "All they did," Florence recalled, "was come and put a card on the door – a big red card with 'Diphtheria' on it."[19] Despite the authority of medical officials, Florence's mother eventually broke the quarantine and ventured into the backyard. A neighbour approached her and offered a remedy for Florence's illness. "She [the neighbour] came over and she had a big white feather – a chicken feather – and a bottle of brandy," recalled Florence, "and she came over and she painted all my tonsils and the inside of my mouth with it ... my mother said it just brought new life to me."[20] As they had done in the case of her polio, Florence's family took advantage of both official and unofficial treatments. Even though professionals warned against the use of any lay treatments, often dismissing them as mere "quackery," many families found them useful and effective. Families were never solely dependent on the wisdom of conventional medical practitioners, nor was professional authority absolute.[21]

MARC

Marc Trapier was born in 1913, five years after Florence. He was one of twelve children and grew up in Hochelaga-Maisonneuve, a working-class suburb on the east end of Montreal, bordering the St Lawrence River.[22] Hochelaga, incorporated into the city of Montreal in the late 1800s, was an industry town with a history of labour unrest. It had a cotton mill, a tobacco factory, and a meat-packing plant and was the site of the first work stoppage in Canada, initiated by female workers at the mill.[23] Although Marc had some fond memories of a tight-knit Catholic Quebecois upbringing, life in Hochelaga was hard. In relation to Montreal, Marc recalled, Hochelaga marked "the barrier for poor people ... it was the slum of the city ... We had running water but electricity was just starting ... When I was seven years old and started school, we had an oil lamp that we would put on the table after the meal and we would sit all around to do our homework."[24] Marc's mother worked at the cotton mill and his father was a blacksmith. He remembered that conforming to social standards of hygiene took both time and energy:

> To have a bath you had to put the boiler on the stove and the stove was not gas but wood. You had to carry the boiled water and put it in the bathtub and we would wash one after another with the same water. It was too hard to get fresh water all over again. And so you would wash four or five kids and the water would be so dirty.[25]

Even in the broader community, he remembered, it was difficult to measure up to ideal standards of public health. "Let's say that you go to the grocery, you buy some rice, you buy some beans, you have to go through everything to remove the – not rats – the mice, all the manure of the mice, you had to clean all that, you have remove it before you cook it ... because in the grocery they would have everything in bowls, you know, and so you had all of those visitors."[26] In Montreal at the turn of the century, like the rest of Quebec, provision of health services was tied closely to religious and ethnic affiliation with French Catholics, English Catholics, Protestants, and Jewish communities providing health services and charitable support to their separate constituencies.[27]

The changing seasons greatly affected family fortunes, Marc recalled, particularly in terms of eating habits and physical comfort. Winter was marked by the constant need to replenish the family's wood supply in order to keep their house adequately heated. It was also the season that demanded his mother's frugality in the kitchen. Marc remembers her formidable negotiating skills at the butcher shop, arguing for the biggest, and cheapest, cuts of meat to feed a large family. She would remove the bone from large cuts of meat and stuff it with whatever root vegetables she had. Despite his mother's efforts, Marc recalls seasonal bouts of hunger.

At the end of the long winter, Marc's mother gave the children their "spring tonic": a concoction of molasses and sulphur familiar to many children in early twentieth-century Canada. Marc recalled it was taken twice a day over a nine-day period and promised to replenish the body's depleted supply of iron and to purify the blood.[28] The warm summer months brought a reprieve from the constant gathering of wood and instead meant a relative bounty of fresh, affordable fruits and vegetables. These were sold door-to-door by merchants pushing carts. Marc didn't look at the calendar during the summer recess from school, preferring instead to mark the passing months by the appearance of strawberries, raspberries, and blueberries. When the merchants offered their first cobs of corn for sale, he knew it was soon time to return to school for another year.[29]

The 1918 flu pandemic struck the Trapier family as it did others in the country and around the world.[30] Although his father and brother were spared and continued to provide for the family when many others lost their main breadwinner, all the other members of the family contracted the flu. Marc was only six years old at the time. His nineteen-year-old brother looked after the daily needs of his siblings and mother while his father worked to provide for the family. Marc recalled that his father took a spoonful of coal oil every morning to fight against the infection. He was convinced that it was this ritual that allowed his father to avoid the flu.[31] Coal oil, often mixed with molasses or sugar, was a common "cure all" home remedy thought to prevent everything from typhoid fever to serious infections to acne.[32]

During his illness, Marc was aware that he was seriously sick because he got to stay in his pajamas for the entire day. He also recalls looking out his window to the street below and seeing grocery carts filled with corpses, victims of the flu, being pushed to the local church. The bodies, however, were not allowed inside. "The priest," he said, "wouldn't let the corpses go into the church because of the influenza ... they used to come out and put some blessed water on them and then they would be put straight into the graves." Memories of his family's concerted efforts to survive the influenza epidemic have long lingered in Marc's consciousness over the years. "It is not easily forgotten," he said.[33] Like the experience of impoverished and working-class families in Winnipeg, as Esyllt Jones has shown, the influenza epidemic struck those with limited means and resources the hardest and with the most devastating consequences.[34]

Equally vivid in Marc's recollections was the sadness experienced through the illness and death of his younger sister. "My sister that was four years younger than me got diphtheria when she was about six or seven years old," Marc recounted. "Her head was just like a ball of fire ... she was suffering, suffering, suffering like mad you know ... and she could not even sleep." She recovered from diphtheria but eventually contracted tuberculosis at the age of fourteen. Marc recalls his mother seating his sister outside the family apartment on a lawn chair to breath in fresh air. Family legend suggests that one of the millionaire owners of the cotton mill where Marc's mother worked saw his sister sitting on the lawn and offered to rent his country cottage to the family to facilitate her convalescence. Unfortunately, they never got the opportunity to take him up on his offer. Marc managed to avoid the disease that eventually ended his sister's life, but he suffered through the trauma associated with losing someone he deeply loved.[35]

The loss of important people in Marc's young life did not end with the death of his sister. When he was eleven, his father, then in his fifty-first year, died of alcoholism.

Three years after his father died, Marc, at the age of 14, began to work full time. A year later he contracted scarlet fever and was quarantined for over a month in a special hospital run by Catholic nuns. Given the increased responsibilities in his life, he recalled his time in the hospital as a welcome respite. "You know, it was the best time of your life! You could have good meals ... the nuns were looking after you."[36]

Marc's childhood struggles with ill health were worsened by the conditions of poverty and deprivation his family endured. In Quebec, religious and ethnic divisions reflected inequities in the provision of health and welfare services. Wealthy, English-speaking Protestants in

Montreal, for example, "created, supported, and managed an array of English-language health facilities and social services to which anglophone skilled and unskilled workers had access."[37] The charity meted out by the Catholic nuns was critical to the survival of Marc's family but it paled in comparison to what wealthier English-speaking Protestants could expect. It was hardly in keeping with broader claims amongst medical professionals about the importance of preventative health services in the fight against contagious diseases in the early decades of the twentieth century.

With similarities to and important differences from the experience of Florence, Marc recalled struggles around health issues as a "family affair." Florence's family, however, remained relatively healthy and free from the life-threatening encounters that plagued the Trapiers. Instead, her family concentrated their energies on combating her polio. Both children recalled encounters with professional medicine in the form of hospitalization and quarantine, but whereas Florence endured these interventions reluctantly, Marc appreciated their possibility for rest and respite. His impoverished working-class experience meant that any unpleasantness around hospitalization and quarantine was tempered by the rest and good food that he enjoyed while under care. This was particularly true for Marc as he was expected to work full time in order to support the family. Conventional attitudes that cast naturalized childhood as free from the concerns and responsibilities of adulthood were often compromised by class constraints and never held true for all children.

ALICE

Alice Mercer was born in 1916 in Montreal in what she described as "a normal household."[38] Seemingly unaware of her privilege compared to children like Marc, she and her brother were raised in an Anglo-Celtic, middle-class family in the north end of the city. Her father was an insurance agent with the Metropolitan Life Insurance Company and her mother, as Alice said, "stayed at home of course – in those days mothers did."[39] Her mother ensured that her children had a hearty breakfast before they headed off to school. "Oh I didn't get out of the house without breakfast. You had to have breakfast. Usually it was oatmeal – porridge ... and toast and jam and marmalade and stuff. Bacon and eggs on weekends."[40] In sharp contrast to the relative deprivation that Marc suffered, Alice remembers abundant, nutritious meals and school lunches:

> We were well-off and we never wanted for anything. She'd [Alice's mother] cook roast lamb. I can remember her roast lamb. And, ah, then she'd make a stew with the other part of the lamb. And we would have stew. And if she had roast beef – usually a rump roast. I remember that from way back. And, ah, she liked to bake and she'd make jam – all kinds of jam every summer ... But, ah, just a normal household.[41]

Despite her privilege, Alice suffered through bouts of common childhood diseases and infections: measles, chicken pox, and scarlet fever. Routine, preventative vaccination against measles and chicken pox, and a host of other diseases and infections, such as rubella and mumps, would be common practice in Canada by the 1960s. In this early period, however, vaccination was routinely contested. Still limited to fighting smallpox, vaccination was often ineffective and caused adverse side effects, including infection from unsanitary procedures. During the smallpox epidemic in the late 1880s, citizens opposed to the compulsory administration of vaccination rioted in the streets of Montreal.[42]

It was her bout with scarlet fever at the age of seven in the early 1920s, however, that caused Alice the most discomfort. Scarlet fever develops as a result of a streptococcus infection and leaves the body particularly susceptible to secondary infections. In the midst of dealing with the scarlet fever, Alice developed abscesses in the jaw area, behind each of her back molar teeth. "I know my mother said I wouldn't have had these abscesses if I had stayed in bed. But I wouldn't stay in bed; I kept getting out of bed." In an era before antibiotics were widely available to kill such disease-causing bacteria, surgical intervention, for those who could afford it, was the best treatment option and, indeed, this is the route that Alice and her family took. After the surgery, Alice remembered a period of daily visits to Montreal's Homeopathic Hospital, eventually renamed Queen Elizabeth Hospital in 1951, to have the area cleaned and gauze dressing changed:

> It was a nice little hospital – even then. It was the Queen E. afterwards. It was the "homeopathetic" we called it – homeopathic [*laughs*]. But, ah, well I didn't mind going. They were very nice to me. I was blond, and I guess they were all reminded of Lillian Gish, I can remember. So I didn't seem to mind.[43]

Alice's hospital visits with her mother were never worrisome or scary. In fact, she looked forward to the daily ritual. "I always got a treat when we were coming home ... ice cream," she said, "if I behaved myself."[44]

The positive hospital experience stood in sharp contrast to a trip to the dentist following the initial misdiagnosis of her infection-induced abscesses. "That [dentist visit] wasn't a very happy experience ... I mean he took my tooth out and it really hurt like heck! ... I can remember yelling at him!" she said.[45] Alice's experience was not unique. In the early decades of the twentieth century, many Canadian children suffered from extremely poor dental hygiene. Doctors, nurses, school medical staff, and public health officials reminded children and their parents of the importance of good nutrition and daily teeth brushing as preventative health strategies.[46] Public health nurses pointed out that for poor families, preventative strategies were often out of their reach. Toothbrushes, toothpaste, as well as nutritionally balanced meals were luxuries few could afford. Blatant bribery, one public health nurse admitted, was a popular way to encourage children to focus attention on their teeth:

> Well, their [children's] love of a bargain often solves the problem: e.g., they can easily be persuaded to clean their teeth regularly when the nurse offers them a large tube of tooth paste and a tooth brush for only ten cents each; or they willingly submit to go to a Dentist when she tells them she will cure the warts of every boy who will have his teeth filled.[47]

Seen as a very last resort, visits to the dentist were to be avoided. As Alice's experience exemplifies, this was based on the fact that anesthetics and painkillers for dental use were neither consistently available nor effective.[48]

Like Marc and Florence, Alice has vivid memories of her mother's home remedies, despite the scorn such approaches received from medical professionals. The Christmas goose, for example, yielded grease that would be rubbed on chests and backs to treat colds. A piece of brown paper would be put overtop of the grease and "you wore that until it practically fell off," Alice fondly remembered.[49] Her mother's homemade cough syrup, made of lemon, glycerine, and syrup of squills, was both effective and pleasant to drink. Mustard plasters were also commonly applied to chests and backs to relieve congestion. Although many of her friends wore small bags of camphor around their necks to ward off seasonal sickness, Alice never did. Her mother rejected this home remedy as pure "superstition."[50]

The Depression years brought a downturn in Alice's father's insurance business, but certainly did not ruin the economic fortunes of the family. Her parents had not invested in the stock market and managed to weather the leaner years. More vividly recalled was her mother's hospitalization in 1929 after she had broken her hip. Alice was twelve years old at the time. She remembers visiting her mother during her eleven-week stay in the same Homeopathic Hospital where her abscess surgery had taken place years before. "She was in a ward with an awful lot of beds," said Alice. "But she was well looked after and she got along well."[51] Born just three years after Marc in the same city, Alice's memories bring into bold relief the pivotal difference that class, ethnicity, and religion made to experiences of healthy living and illness in childhood. While medical professionals promoted a shift from an emphasis on the treatment of contagious diseases to their prevention in these early decades, its potential benefits applied only selectively.

THERESA

Theresa Elliott was born in 1920 in the countryside around Parry Sound, Ontario – a town much smaller than Vancouver or Montreal – to a lower middle-class, Anglo-Celtic family. The family had seven children – four girls and three boys – Theresa was the oldest. Her father was a general contractor and worked with lumber while her mother worked at home, supporting the children. Theresa recalled a happy home life in which religious faith provided a guiding set of principles for the family. She recalled growing up during the Depression years as neither-well off and completely immune to its effects, nor impoverished and hungry. "No," she said. "We were just your average family in the Depression."[52]

At twenty-one months, two years before her next sibling came along, Theresa became ill. Her parents brought her into Parry Sound on the local train to see the doctor. By the time she arrived at his office, Theresa was running a very high fever and had stiffness in her muscles. The doctor was unable to diagnose her condition. He sought permission from Theresa's parents for exploratory surgery, although Theresa could not recall why he thought this would be a useful course of action. Her parents refused to give consent. Instead, they decided that Theresa should be taken to Toronto's Hospital for Sick Children for examination and diagnosis. Unlike Florence Drake a decade before her, Theresa's parents were skeptical of their local doctor's approach and opted instead to seek what they hoped was more sophisticated treatment in the city. Like Florence Drake, however, Theresa was eventually diagnosed with poliomyelitis, also known as infantile paralysis, the first such case in the Parry Sound district, according to her family.[53] Despite the clear diagnosis, however, the success of treatment held no guarantee for her improvement. The family returned home to Parry Sound with instructions to lay Theresa on boards to try to prevent possible curvature of the spine.

During her early days of home treatment, Theresa's health was extremely unstable. "I was either too sick, or not sick and getting better!" she recalled. An army nurse who lived nearby offered to assist Theresa's mother with treatment. She was familiar with the Sister Kenny method, developed over the course of the First World War by an Australian army nurse, Elizabeth Kenny.[54] It wasn't until the 1920s, however, that Kenny's controversial method of messaging and exercising the limbs of polio victims, instead of the conventional method of applying plaster casts, gained widespread approval and use. Thus, in the initial months of living with polio, Theresa recalled long periods of time during which her mother and the nurse put warm olive oil on her legs, wrapped them in wool blankets, and massaged them. Despite these rigorous attempts to improve her mobility, Theresa remained completely paralyzed. On the ninth day of massage treatment, however, she reached up and grabbed her mother's hand. That moment marked a long and slow journey towards improved, although never complete, mobility.[55] The family's distance from a major hospital clearly had ramifications for Theresa's mother. Charged with providing physical therapy for her daughter was simply added to the other duties of caring for a growing family.

The family coped as best they could with Theresa's limited mobility. When she was four years old, she developed enough muscle capacity to walk upright and without assistance. Before that, and with the constant concern of her mother, she did what she could to help herself. "I was mostly creeping. Yeah, I had to start all over again. There mainly seemed to be more cuddling, and Mom was scared that it would come back again, and she was over-protective. And they – I was four before she had another child which gave mother a break."[56]

Like Florence years before her, Theresa was fitted with special braces to support her underdeveloped leg that she wore only at night. It was not something that bothered her or made her uncomfortable, she recalled. She was young and simply accepted it as "normal."

Like Florence, Marc, and Alice, Theresa has vivid memories of home remedies and tonics made by her mother. Theresa took a similar sulphur and molasses tonic each spring as Marc had done. Her mother baked onions sprinkled with brown sugar in the oven and served the juice from them to the children. This was believed to ward off winter colds. The baked and softened onion would then be hung around the neck as a kind of poultice. Theresa's mother was also adamant that the children wash their hands with a special "red soap." "We didn't use Lux or anything like that. She had this one certain kind – it was disinfecting, and I know some of the kids in the school would have impetigo, and none of us would have it because my mother used this disinfectant soap."[57]

Despite the precautionary hand washing and preventative tonic drinking, the major childhood diseases still managed to infect the Elliott family. When Theresa was seven or eight, the family found themselves quarantined. One by one, each of the seven Elliott children developed the telltale symptoms of measles: high fevers and the characteristic rash associated with this highly contagious viral respiratory infection. When the local health officer visited the family after the allotted time to decide whether or not the quarantine could be lifted, Theresa's mother begged the children to look as perky and recovered as they could. "We are going to get that quarantine off one way or another!" Theresa's mother had vowed. She was clearly desperate to ensure that it was lifted and normal life resumed. To the delight and relief of the entire family, the "quarantine" sign left with the health officer.[58] The concerted efforts on the part of the Elliott family to have the quarantine lifted echoes the desperation that led Florence's mother to break their quarantine years before. The medical imperative to contain and prevent the spread of contagion was often completely incompatible and unsustainable in the context of the pressures of family life in the early decades of the twentieth century.[59]

The challenge of Theresa's mobility was not, however, a temporary proposition. She did not attend school regularly until she was ten years old. Theresa attributed this to the fact of her polio and her inability to keep her balance, particularly during the winter months when snow and ice made conditions treacherous for walking. By the time she was ten, however, Theresa desperately wanted to attend school as regularly as possible. She started in the first grade. "I really worked hard 'cause there were kids four years younger than I was in the same class. And I really worked hard. And I went right through to the ninth grade. I passed the ninth grade and I went right through in six years. I skipped two classes twice."[60]

Theresa walked with a pronounced limp during her childhood but did not recall any teasing or poor treatment from her school peers. In fact, her peers accommodated her differences with ease. As Theresa recalled,

> I had a very happy life, and I was considered along with the rest of them. I never heard any of them saying, "You can't do this or

you can't do that" ... And I remember when we played ball, we were twelve years of age and I was wonderful at hitting the baseball. And my teammates would say, "That's fine Theresa, you strike the ball, and I'll run for you." And that's how they treated me.[61]

This accommodating approach was not something that Theresa felt she really needed, despite her gratitude for it. At home, she remembered, she was treated the same as her other siblings. "I had to plug along with the rest of them," she recalled. In the care of a supportive family and extended network of neighbours and classmates, Theresa's disability was managed relatively successfully.

As Theresa began to gain more mobility in her pre-teen years, the family returned to the HSC hoping for more treatment options. Once again, however, they were disappointed:

They [the doctors] told me they couldn't do anything for me. They didn't know anything about this infantile paralysis, but I had come out of the critical part of it and I didn't have the fever. And it left me completely – on the right side – I have a smaller leg and a smaller hip, but they said they couldn't do anything for me.[62]

The family was encouraged to wait until Theresa was sixteen years old to return to Toronto for a series of operations on her leg. Her parents dutifully heeded this advice and Theresa has very vivid memories of this time. At this point, she was too old to be a patient at HSC, so she was admitted to a ward at the Toronto General Hospital. She recalls that there were twenty-eight beds in her ward. She was the youngest patient. "Everyone on the ward called me 'Snooks,' and I was in there three times – I had to go back – and I had a cast put on, and then I went home for two months, and then I went back and that went on for two years," she recalled. Hospital staff insisted that she and other young polio patients develop a positive attitude in order to overcome physical limitations. She remembered,

When I went to Toronto when I was sixteen, they drilled into me that, "Your polio is in your mind. You can do anything. Don't let your polio keep you down." ... And I remember one girl had polio in both legs, and they stood her up against the wall and she walked with these crutches. And they say to her, "Come on Doreen, you got to walk." [She would say] "I can't." She'd cry and she would cry. And do you know before she left the hospital, she was walking. But they found – that was our therapy – it's in our mind, that we can do it.[63]

Theresa's memories suggest that she was often caught between the power of positive (and individualized) thinking to improve herself and societal prejudice that constrained that improvement. Like Florence Drake, Theresa believed that her disability ultimately forced her out of the (highly gendered) dating and marriage economy that preoccupied her non-disabled peers. She decided to become a missionary to Africa as a worthy alternative vocation for her future. "I never regret being lame – never," she confided. "In fact, I said that I would never marry ... I was going to Africa. I was going to be a missionary. I was bound I was going to go to Africa ... because I never thought that anybody – down deep in my heart I never thought that anybody would take me because I was lame. I had that idea."[64] Theresa cancelled her missionary plans when she met Richard, who would eventually become her husband. She recalled that he encouraged her to downplay and ignore her physical differences:

And even after I got married, I went out and I cut the lawn. And my husband came home and I said, "Look it, I bet the neighbours are talking away about me out there limping away and cutting that lawn." And he said, "Why? There's nothing wrong with you." And he would never, never say to me, "Well you can't do that." He encouraged me.[65]

When Theresa suggested that she use the brace and shoe that she wore as a young girl for a planter in her garden, Richard balked. "My husband wouldn't allow it," she confided with a chuckle.[66]

CONCLUSIONS

In the early decades of the twentieth century, health professionals prioritized the containment and eradication of contagious diseases through improved public health and medicalized interventions. With the rise of pediatric medicine, as detailed in chapter 1, the message to families was to increase their engagement with professional practitioners in order to prevent childhood illness. This message of detection and prevention was circulated through child welfare clinics, public health practitioners, and school nurses. Reporting on her experiences as a school nurse in Regina in 1911, Jean Browne nicely summarized the need for health surveillance in schools in dramatic terms:

> The trouble seems to have been that, in the zeal for stuffing Johnny with useful knowledge, people forget that he was an animal before he was man ... they drove him into the school house where he acquired, with almost equal certainty, mathematics and mumps, spelling and sore throat, grammar and grippe.[67]

The childhood memories explored in this chapter provide another lens on these professional priorities, fine tuning our understanding of how children and families experienced ill health during these early decades. Many Canadian children over the course of the twentieth century contracted, lived with, or died as a result of the childhood diseases that affected Florence, Marc, Alice, and Theresa. The germ theory of disease transmission was well established by the early years of the twentieth century and with it came admonitions from multiple quarters – public health officials, doctors, nurses, and educators – for the observance of hygienic science. Cleanliness, particularly hand washing, and (at least) weekly baths, the use of a regularly laundered handkerchief, plenty of fresh air, and moderate exercise were recommended as part of a healthy regime.[68] As the histories recounted here suggest, however, constraints associated with daily living made easy compliance with such idealized advice difficult, if not impossible. Each participant recalled their parents' – particularly their mothers' – engagement with domestic doctoring, albeit in varying degrees and regardless of class affiliation. They drew on a mixture of folk and professional wisdom to treat their children's pain and/or discomfort. Medical and public health professionals certainly wielded influence, but they were far from the only purveyors of treatment.

While the impact of race emerges more clearly in the memories of the adults explored in the next chapter, the constraints and opportunities associated with class, ethnicity, and gender are clearly evident here. The parents of Florence, Alice, and Theresa drew upon their extra resources to respond to threats against their daughters' health. Whether they paid out of pocket or took advantage of external resources offered or known to them, consultation with medical professionals augmented, but didn't necessarily supplant familial responses to illness. In an era before socialized medicine and despite the challenges disease epidemics posed for all families, survival for working-class, French Canadian families like the Trapiers was more difficult. When epidemic diseases struck, those with little financial security could scarcely afford either the cost of professional care or the loss of a wage earner, including youngsters. At the age of fourteen, Marc was a full-time worker. That his time in a Catholic charity quarantine hospital with scarlet fever was remembered as a welcomed respite from work and hunger underscored the significant difference class made to children's experiences. Of the girls, only Florence worked for pay while she was a teenager. At the age of seventeen, and even though she had not applied for the job, she became a telephone switchboard operator at the request of one of the telephone company's owners.[69] Unlike Marc's experience, neither frequent nor even occasional bouts of hunger characterized the girls' middle-class childhoods. Lack of adequate, nutritious food may have seriously undermined Marc's ability, and that of his family, to escape sickness and death. In sharp contrast, food was abundant and its enjoyment a "normal" part of childhood for the girls.

A short time after the death of his father, Marc was expected to work. This was in keeping with gendered constraints that dictated that men, even boys, naturally engaged in waged labour when circumstances warranted. Gendered constraints also had a profound impact on the experience of Florence and Theresa, both of whom keenly felt its power to exclude. The effects of polio left both women with physical disabilities and, given rigid codes of feminine beauty, largely outside mainstream adolescent culture.

The memories of Florence, Marc, Alice, and Theresa establish that health concerns were first and foremost familial concerns shaped in large part by social circumstances. Bouts of epidemic disease and chronic illness took on differing meanings within different families and had a profound impact upon family routines and strategies for survival. While professional practitioners were key figures in the memories of the participants, the authority they wielded varied from family to family. In this early period, professional help was sought out after other, perhaps more affordable and effective avenues were explored. When serious illnesses struck as it did in the childhood memories of all four participants, families had to strategize, compromise, and cope in order to survive.

3

Shirley, Lily, Jack, and Lina: Healthy Bodies and Domestic Doctoring, 1920s to the 1940s

The interwar decades saw the strengthening and consolidation of a number of public health initiatives aimed at improving the health and welfare of Canadian families. Efforts to improve infant and maternal health, such as the introduction of well-baby clinics and milk pasteurization depots, helped lower infant mortality rates over the period, but tenacious gaps between upper- and lower-income families prevailed.[1] In 1926, a vaccine against diphtheria was made available. By the end of the Second World War, inoculations against small pox had all but successfully ended widespread epidemics of the virulent killer.[2] The addition of fluoride to municipal water supplies slowly began in an effort to improve dental health. Just as compulsory vaccination had sparked controversy in an earlier period, however, fluoridation was contested in many communities where doubt about its efficacy endured.[3] In 1937, signaling at least ostensibly the entrenchment of medical doctors as leading experts in health provision, the Royal College of Physicians and Surgeons of Canada formally recognized pediatrics as a free-standing medical specialty.[4]

In all provinces except Quebec and Newfoundland, compulsory school attendance was increasingly enforced for both rural and urban children. Many schools throughout the country developed medical inspections, hired school doctors and nurses, and ran dental clinics. In some small and remote communities, schools represented the only site of regular, albeit often inadequate, medical attention. Fraught as it was with superficial, incomplete, or incompetent medical services, school medical inspection made some headway towards detecting and treating children's ailments before they escalated into more serious health challenges.⁵ The entrenchment of professional medical authority over the health of children, evidenced by the growth of public health infrastructure and the curricular inclusion of health in public education over the interwar period, emboldened practitioners to demand and expect total compliance from parents. The faith placed in the equation of good health with a happy, successful life was absolute. In rather turgid prose, the authors of *Health Essentials for Canadian Schools* (1938), prescribed for use in British Columbian schools, exemplified this attitude:

> Health is a pearl of great price. Illness and physical defects frequently involve discomfort, pain, expense, inefficiency, failure, and discouragement. Good health on the contrary makes for physical and mental vigour, greater ease in learning, the acquisition of property, the improvement of one's personal appearance, social approval, success, and happiness.⁶

The oral histories of Shirley, Lily, Jack, and Lina, like those in the previous chapter, enrich and complicate straightforward narratives of medical progress over the twentieth century. Their experiences remind us that alongside efforts on the part of medical professionals to entrench their dominance in areas of health and well-being, families continued to provide their own medical care and attention. Doctors, nurses, teachers, and school medical staff provided important services, but "good health" was also very much shaped by the exigencies of race, class, and gender.

SHIRLEY

Born in 1924, Shirley Brand spent the early part of her childhood growing up on a First Nation reserve in Deseronto, Ontario. Her mother, a Chippewa, found herself unhappy living with her husband's family and longed to return to her own in Alderville, Ontario. Eventually the marriage broke down and Shirley remained with her father, of Mohawk and English descent, and his extensive network of sisters, aunts, uncles, and grandparents. As Shirley fondly remembered,

> I used to go and live with all these aunts and uncles. And they were all my grandmother's brothers and sisters and when my dad was working I guess everybody took turns looking after me. I never missed out ... they were all so good to me. I remember my early childhood as being very happy. I had good parents and I had good relatives. When my mother left, I never missed her because I had so many loving aunts. I can't remember ever being sad. Everybody was fussing over me.[7]

With the exception of a cold or two, Shirley managed to escape the typical diseases of childhood – chicken pox, measles, mumps – that afflicted others. Her grandmother, like Alice's mother a decade before, treated colds with goose grease rubbed on the back and camphor salts wafted under the nose. Both treatments, although unpleasant, resulted in improved health, Shirley recalled.[8]

Given the difficulties of finding steady employment during the Depression years, particularly for First Nations peoples, Shirley and her father greatly benefited from a wide circle of supportive family. Her father caught white fish at the Bay of Quinte and sold his catch from a cart on the reserve. In conjunction with plentiful fishing, relatives hunted duck and often ate communally. Shirley recalled large duck hunting parties at the beach at Quinte where "the women would be on the beach, and the men would shoot the ducks and then the women would clean them and then they would have a big feast."[9]

Shirley lived on the Deseronto reserve until she was around eight years old. As she shared her memories of growing up, she reflected on the wide gap between popular images of reservation life and what she remembered about her experiences:

> I can't ever remember, like when I look at pictures on television of these reservations, I can't associate my childhood with that – with feather hats and the beating drums and all that stuff. I can't see that we were any different than we are today. Well we are more modern today, but in those days like I mean I lived with an aunt – my father's aunt, and she had a nice home, she was a great cook, and they lived on a farm, grew all their own vegetables.

Some of Shirley's most vivid childhood memories involve her mixed experiences at the Deseronto reserve day school that was staffed by non-Aboriginal teachers and located across the street from her home. During her first day of school, she decided that it was not for her ("'Boy,' I thought, 'I don't like it here!'") and she promptly walked home. Shirley's dad brought her back to school. The next day, however, she did the same thing. Over time, she stayed at school for longer and longer periods, growing to enjoy it immensely. She also recalled that the non-Aboriginal "lady teacher" would occasionally take her to her home, give her dinner, wash her hair and set it into curls. "I think she did that because I had no mother," Shirley explained.[10] Alongside racial and class-based assumptions about what constituted a "normal" or "good" childhood, the teacher's actions, particularly setting Shirley's hair in curls, also conveyed gendered assumptions about proper girlhood.

Between the ages of eight and twelve, Shirley moved three times as her father searched for steady work. Shannonville, a community nine miles west of Deseronto, was their home for one year. Despite their brief time there, a particular memory from her school experience stayed with Shirley. For many families without the convenience of heated running water, bath time was limited to a weekly ritual. This was common practice in an earlier time period, as the previous chapter makes clear, and for many rural communities such amenities continued to be absent well into the twentieth century.[11] "There was this boy in the school who was very, very dirty," Shirley recalled. "And you know, I thought the most humiliating thing when I grew older – the teacher couldn't stand it so she got a tub of water and we would all takes turns washing him – his back and his hair ... he had his underwear on ..." She speculated that the teacher was making an example of this particular boy, using the power of public humiliation to encourage him to bathe more often. The only lasting impression it had on her, however, was confusion, regret, and sadness: "That was a really awful thing to do to him – so embarrassing. And yet maybe he wasn't embarrassed. I don't know."[12]

In 1933, a job opportunity picking fruit in Grimsby meant that Shirley and her father moved again. Shirley's father remarried and although her stepmother was kind and tried to provide support, her efforts were neither wanted nor appreciated. "As the years went on I grew to appreciate her," Shirley regretfully recalled. "But it was only that age. I mean she tried to do everything for me, and I never realized – well at the time I didn't want her to do anything for me, and I didn't want to talk to her even."[13]

In 1936, the family moved to Kearney, Ontario. Shirley was twelve years old. She recalled that the local doctor and his wife offered "facts of life" talks to the young girls of the community. While Shirley thought this was useful and necessary, her stepmother was appalled and suspicious of the offer. "He got in touch with the girls my age that were at the school and he wanted us to go to his house so he could explain the facts of life to us, because he knew that people weren't doing that," she remembered. "And of course my stepmother was upset about that. She thought he had no business talking about that to young girls." Precisely what motivated the local doctor to provide this information, beyond professional duty and benevolence, was never made clear to Shirley. While very much in keeping with gendered expectations that relegated girls to the role of sexual gatekeepers, frank discussion of sex and sexuality were largely taboo subjects, most particularly outside the private boundaries of the family. Even within families, the topic of sexuality and the physical changes brought on by puberty was broached rarely and tentatively.[14] Nevertheless, Shirley attended one session offered by the doctor and his wife, along with five or six of her female classmates. Her stepmother was vehemently opposed, however, and Shirley's participation did not continue. As events in her life unfolded, this missed opportunity, however complicated, was prescient. As she entered her teenaged years in Kearney, Shirley recalled stark instances in which racism and sexism made their unwelcome presence keenly felt. "There were boys who made fun of me," she recalled. "They would call me 'squaw' and that used to really embarrass me." She found herself confused and unsettled by intimate heterosexual dating, even as her father encouraged her relationship with one young man. "I mean I couldn't discuss it [dating and sexuality] with anybody and I think I was so uninformed that I just didn't know how to accept that sexual part," Shirley said. Her first sexual experience with the young man favoured by her father resulted in an unplanned pregnancy. In 1941, seventeen-year-old Shirley married and shortly afterwards gave birth to twins.[15] They weighed only four pounds combined. Shirley struggled to feed the babies and despite constant vigilance and support from the women in her community, she lost Marian when she was three months old. The other twin, Trina, was rushed to Toronto's Hospital for Sick Children and remained there for six months. Eventually, Trina was diagnosed as severely lactose intolerant. After the diagnosis and a switch to a special formula, Trina was discharged, returned home, and thrived under the care of her grateful mother:

> And when she was nine months old, we went and got her. And she only weighed nine pounds, but she was so bright. And she couldn't digest regular milk ... And, ah, I used to have to make a formula. But she came along. She put on the weight left, right, and centre, and she was just a healthy normal kid by the time she reached two. And so we were just so thankful to have her.[16]

It was difficult to be a teenager and a young wife and mother, Shirley remembered. But she also recalled that her supportive First Nation community enabled her family to cope and thrive. "When I look back," she concluded, "I look with fond memories and I think that I am fortunate."[17]

LILY

Lily Mason was born in Fort Pelly, Saskatchewan in 1925. Of First Nation ancestry, she grew up in the company of her parents, four brothers, and two sisters. She recalled a happy childhood, albeit one circumscribed by poverty. They had a quarter section farm on 160 acres of rocky and swampy land given to her father for military service during the First World War. It was largely unsuitable for large-scale cultivation. What little land they could use supported a few horses, cows, oats, and some vegetables. Potatoes, the main stable of the winter months, turnips, carrots, peas, beans, and squash rounded out her childhood diet. Lily grew up in what she described as "a little two-room shack ... a kitchen and a bedroom ... the boys slept in the kitchen and we [Lily and her sister] shared the bedroom with our mom and dad with a curtain between us ... tight quarters ... oh were they ever."[18]

The provision of adequate food, particularly through the harsh Saskatchewan winters, was a constant struggle. Hard times for the family were accentuated during the Depression years. At the worst of times, Lily recalled surviving on little more than potatoes stored in the root cellar and bread. Her father was a skilled hunter and fisher, however, and managed as best he could to feed his large family:

> He would hang it [meat] up in the fir trees outside high enough so the animals wouldn't get at it. And once in a while we were supplemented with fish 'cause he had a fish route for couple of winters that I remember. He would go up to Lake Manitoba to a little village there and pick up a load of fish, and then he had his fish day pack and then he had his route where he would drop off orders for fish at the different places, and what was left over, he brought home and stored in the snow bank. That was the only refrigeration available at that time.[19]

Birth and death punctuated many of Lily's most vivid childhood memories. When she was around four years of age, her five-month-old baby brother died of what the coroner characterized as "double pneumonia." Although he had always had trouble breathing throughout his short life (his chest "rattled all the time"), Lily's mother attributed the baby's death to the ineptitude of a substitute midwife. Lily stated emphatically:

> Not our regular midwife, who was a wonderful woman and she delivered the rest of us safely, but on this occasion she was sick or busy elsewhere. Anyways, she couldn't come for his birth. Another woman came instead. And I think she bungled it 'cause she [Lily's mother] said he must have breathed in fluid into his lungs after he was born.[20]

The venerated midwife, who was also a medicine woman, Lily recalled, had safely delivered hundreds of babies in the area. This record was attributed in large part to the meticulous standards of cleanliness the medicine woman adhered to. "I remember her sterilizing ripped open flour sacks that had been washed and boiled and, ah, she would use these during the delivery," Lily said. "Now what she used them for, I don't know." The midwife also sterilized the moss that Lily's mother gathered as a natural absorbent to be used during the birth.[21]

The midwife/medicine woman was not only adept at handling an impeding birth, as Lily and her siblings learned first-hand at the time of her younger sister's arrival. Lily recalled that while her mother was in labour, the medicine woman gave her and her older siblings a black tea to drink. Each child was instructed to take only a few sips of the tea. "It had a rather pleasant taste," Lily remembered, "and it knocked us all out at the same time ... we woke up the next morning at nine o'clock all at the same time and we had a new sister there."[22] Clearly, the medicine woman understood the necessity for Lily's mother to give birth in peace and to have some precious time to rest undisturbed by her other curious and demanding children.

The midwife/medicine woman limited her practice to childbirth. This, according to Lily, kept her so busy that other kinds of ailments had to be dealt with in the family, by the medicine man, or by a conventional doctor. The family availed themselves of all three options. When her mother became severely ill with pneumonia, the doctor made the seven-mile journey to examine her. In the depths of the Depression, few people could afford to pay the doctor with money. "I think most of his patients around that little town had seldom – well I think he was given food and vegetables and so forth, I think, but there was no actual money because nobody had any money in those days," Lily pointed out. Although the family didn't have to pay for the treatment, they did have to arrange a horse and sleigh to get him to their farm. He visited three times, Lily vividly remembered, which signaled the severity of her mother's affliction. She eventually recovered.[23]

On two occasions, once to drain an abscessed tooth and once to deal with her son's vomiting and diarrhea, Lily's mother sought out the help of the medicine man. Lily remembered that although the "regular doctor" had seen her brother and had prescribed medicine for him, his condition was not improving. Indeed, it was getting worse. "He was so weak," Lily remembered, "that he could barely hold his head up." The medicine man

> crushed up a white root, but when he crushed it up and shook it in a bottle it turned pink. And he told her [Lily's mother] to give him a teaspoon or two of that throughout the day. And by suppertime that night, he was feeling well enough to sit up and bang his spoon on the table [laughs]. So it just took him the one day to recover.[24]

Although Lily managed to escape many of the serious illnesses that plagued her family, she suffered other troublesome and painful health challenges. One of the worst in her experience were excruciating earaches: "They would last pretty near a whole week from the onset of the ache and then the swelling would start and then it would get worse and the whole neck area would be swollen on one side." Two of her siblings suffered similar bouts of ear infections. Lily's mother warmed some of Dr Thomas' Eclectic Oil, purchased along with Zam-Buk salve from the traveling Watkins salesman that visited the farm, and dropped some in the ear.[25] She would then have Lily lie down, resting her ear on a bag of salt that had been warmed up on the stove. This would bring some temporary relief from the throbbing pain. It was remarkable, Lily believed, that she suffered no long-term hearing loss from her painful battles.

Lily recalls that when she developed a case of ringworm on her arm, her mother simply treated her with veterinary supplies. The solution for horses that developed the fungal infection was to rub bluestone, or copper sulfate, on the affected area. A "few dabs" of bluestone were put on Lily's arm. "It was effective because I didn't have it for too long – maybe for about two or three days," she recalled. Although bluestone or blue vitriol was used as an effective fungicide and an emetic, it was also toxic and its medical use, especially for children, eventually fell out of favour.[26]

On at least two occasions the entire family was infested with head lice. Even though head lice never discriminate between clean and dirty hair, there was a significant social stigma associated with it in the experience of some children. "The kids would tease each other about them," Lily recalled. "The children who escaped head lice would needle the other kids who got them."[27] Ridding the family of lice was a labour-intensive and toxic undertaking that typically fell onto mothers. The imperative was to act quickly and decisively to kill each and every one of often hundreds of nits and to prevent re-infestations. Half measures were seldom successful. Lily's mother followed the typical course of action: the children's heads were soaked with kerosene oil and a fine-tooth comb was repeatedly pulled through the hair. After this painful process – the scalp often burning from the kerosene oil – the hair was wrapped in a towel for a number of hours and then shampooed.

Like Shirley, Lily's memories of school were formative in many ways. She attended a one-room schoolhouse located two miles from their home. She remembered the walk to school as rather pleasant during warmer months and something akin to torture during the scathing prairie winters. The school was heated by a basement furnace that pumped heat into the classroom through a large register along the back baseboards. Those who lived closest to the school were expected to show up early and start up the furnace. Her teacher, she recalled, was "excellent ... She managed to get all those kids from grade one to nine through school ... even the children who didn't speak English ... a lot of Russians, Polish, Swedish, Norwegian ... there was the whole United Nations there." While two neighbours could afford cars, most of Lily's school peers travelled by horse-and-sleigh and typically had just enough food to go around. One classmate, she recalled, suffered from the effects of malnutrition: "That little girl was so terribly thin. And, ah, she grew up OK, but I don't think that family – that family had very little to eat, if anything." Her father's winter game hunting was shared around the community. "He divided it up amongst the people who were having a hard time of it ... my parents were good that way," she remembered.[28]

The realities of this Depression-era rural community, however, were far removed from the ideals prescribed by a well-meaning official health curriculum and teacher. Lily was quick to point the chasm between these important influences in her life:

She [Lily's teacher] tried to teach us about – like daily hygiene – like after breakfast brushing your teeth. And I don't think any of the kids in that school owned a toothbrush. I know I didn't until

I was twelve years old ... and what to pack for lunch – her idea of a good lunch was a sandwich, a couple of cookies or a cake, and an orange or an apple, and which most of us only saw once a year at Christmastime.[29]

In other ways, however, Lily suggested that schools presented important opportunities to protect and improve one's health. Yearly visits by a school nurse meant inoculations against major health threats, such as diphtheria and smallpox, could be received without cost. Taking full advantage of free health services offered to the community through the local school was critical to Lily's family and, she believed, made the difference between life and death.[30]

JACK

Jack McCrea was born in Huntsville, Ontario in 1926, one year after Lily. He had one brother, born three years later. Settled in the area since the late 1800s, he was the third generation of the McCrea family to call the area home. His mother's parents divorced when she was eight years old and she decided to immigrate to Canada from Scotland with her father and brother. She never attended school, Jack pointed out, working instead as a maid. During the hard years of the Depression, the McCrea family was better off than most of their neighbours. Benefiting from the economic privilege of the male breadwinner, Jack's father's employment at Huntsville's Anglo-Canadian Leather Company tannery provided the family with some financial security. "We did alright," Jack recalled, "but there was a lot of people in Huntsville that didn't, but my mother would make a great big stew or something, and then she'd – she'd have them all down from up the street ... she fed a lot of kids." Like Lily's family, the McCrea's helped their neighbours through the worst of the Depression years.

Growing up, Jack recalled that his mother was well-known in the community for her skill of tending to the sick and dealing effectively with a variety of ailments. She was often more effective, he affirmed, then the conventional doctor. As Jack recalled,

I think I had the first case in Huntsville of impetigo. The doctor didn't know what it was – it was eating the flesh between my fingers and on my ears ... the doctor bandaged my hands all up and I had to stay out of school and then I'd meet – anybody that met me, they'd cross the street – they didn't want to catch it, I guess. My mother put some Mecca ointment on it and it cured it.³¹

Proud of his mother's accomplishments despite her lack of formal education, Jack pointed out that she never learned to read and write, relying instead on her memory for various healing salves and tonics. "My mother was the doctor on Mary Street," Jack remembered. "Anybody that was having trouble or anything – you'd see her going with her hot water bottle and bottle of castor oil and a teaspoon."³²

While he recalled his father also making home remedies, it was his mother who stood out in this respect. Like many others, the McCreas took advantage of manufactured remedies made available, particularly to rural families, through traveling salesmen. The Rawleigh salesman would come around twice a year with a "couple of great big club bags ... and he had all kinds of medicines in there and salves and stuff for the kitchen ... everybody was happy to see him coming."³³ His mother routinely purchased Rawleigh's ointment for use in her domestic doctoring work. Other remedies, such as camphor bags worn around the neck, mustard plasters that "stayed on you until spring came," wild strawberry elixir, ginger tea, and onion poultices were made and administered by his mother. "And then for whooping cough – a real good remedy was brown sugar and coal oil. That cut the phlegm or something ... she would give you that on a teaspoon," he recalled.³⁴

Head lice infestation was a constant challenge. Like Lily, Jack endured painful sessions in which his coal oil- or kerosene oil-soaked-head was checked meticulously for nits with a fine-tooth comb. He was also affected by the social stigma attached to such an infestation. "Today I still won't go and buy a fine-tooth comb," Jack confided. "Everybody would know you were lousy. And then you got your head washed with soap and coal oil and everything to kill the damn things."³⁵

For all their usefulness, home remedies also had their limitations. When the measles or chicken pox struck, for example, Jack recalled that "you just laid in bed until you got over it ... you could do nothing for it ... Mother just kept us warm ... then when you got over it, you were over it." At the age of eleven, Jack recounted the particularly heartbreaking death of his fourteen-year-old friend and neighbour from pneumonia. He recalled sadly, "the onion poultices didn't do much for him."[36]

Although he recalled a childhood relatively free from major, life-threatening illnesses, Jack's teeth were a particular challenge. He made frequent visits to the dentist and was overjoyed when nitrous oxide became a routinely used anesthetic. Prior to this, and as Alice Mercer's experience a decade earlier testifies, children simply had to endure the pain. The nitrous oxide ("laughing gas") was administered through a mask attached to a long tube with a ball on the end that the patient could squeeze to increase the dose. Jack recalled that the dentist would teasingly accuse him of using up all the gas in one visit! When Jack enlisted in the navy in 1943 at the age of seventeen, like many other young Canadian men he had all his teeth pulled and was fitted with dentures. "I was glad to see them go," he recalled. "They always gave me trouble."[37]

LINA

Lina Colussi was born in Kelowna, British Columbia in 1926 to Italian immigrant parents. The Colussi family came to Canada in 1910 and settled on a farm in the lush Okanagan Valley. Lina was the fifth of seven children born into the family. Only four children, however, survived infancy. Two brothers, including the first- and fourth-born, died shortly after their birth.[38]

Lina enjoyed what she called an "idyllic" childhood. She did not remember being adversely affected by the Depression in ways that so deeply affected Lily's family. In keeping with the lives of others highlighted in this chapter, however, she was surrounded by a very close-knit family and extended community, joined together in her case by their status as immigrants, Italian-Canadians, and members of the Catholic Church. Her parents sponsored other family members who also decided to immigrant to Canada and the Okanagan Valley. "So it was very community-minded," Lina said, "and the Italians had their Italian picnic once or twice a year, and Italian fish farms – so we did all those kinds of cultural things." Measuring her material circumstances through her father's economic standing in the community, Lina recalled,

> Oh, I would say my dad was a very prosperous farmer. You know we weren't, by today's standards, rich, but we certainly weren't poor. We had lots to eat, and my dad had – you know in the thirties – two vehicles – one for the farm – a truck and a car, which was almost unheard of ... everything was quite up-to-date ... we didn't want for anything or need anything ... it was very simple, but we had everything we needed.[39]

Growing up in the Okanagan Valley, located in the southern interior of the province, Lina was raised on what she described as a "typical Italian-Mediterranean" diet. An abundance of food – fresh vegetables, fruits, eggs, chicken, pork, cheese – was always available. Her good fortune in this regard was never taken for granted. Lina was taught that good nutrition was a building block for a healthy life:

> Everybody had a garden. Everybody had chickens in their yard. And everybody did preserves certainly in the dead of winter, especially with my dad having all the fruits and vegetables we ever wanted. We had three or four vegetables everyday; we had fruit everyday. We would have meat, eggs, chicken, pork, and beef. Our diet couldn't have been better, and I am sure this why I have really good skin today, and good hair, and I certainly don't look my age. I think a lot of it is because we grew up on such a healthy diet.[40]

Paralleling the memories of others profiled here, Lina recalled that her mother was a significant provider of home remedies. When diet alone did not prevent illness or disease, she employed prepared medicines purchased twice a year from the "Watkins man" who travelled the Valley. Her mother would also routinely give Lina and her siblings a laxative pill to keep them "regular." She also used simple home remedies. Impetigo was effectively dealt with by administering a mixture of baking soda and water. Reminiscent of

Lily's experience, Lina also recalled that an aching ear would receive a warm drizzle of olive oil.[41]

In 1927, the western provinces, beginning with British Columbia and moving eastward, were hit with the second wave of the poliomyelitis epidemic.[42] One year later, at the age of two, Lina contracted the disease. She was not expected to survive it. "I remember my parents telling me they didn't expect me to live that night," Lina remembered. "There were a lot of young children that did get it. But I pulled through. But at that time, too, there was sort of a lot of stigma to polio, and they also put you in quarantine and disinfected all the houses."[43] While Lina's polio turned out to be a mild case, her family was privileged enough to take advantage of a number of treatment avenues. At the age of three, she spent a year at the Queen Alexandra Solarium in Mill Bay on Vancouver Island, a centre that specialized in heliotherapy, or "sun cure," for treating polio, tuberculosis, and other chronic illnesses.[44] "I don't remember my time there," Lina said, but "the doctor wrote a report almost every month of my progress." Lina does remember that when she returned home, her parents made every effort to continue the treatment protocols begun at the solarium:

> I do remember having to wear braces and the special shoe, and the one thing that my parents always did – they always recommended the massaging and burying your leg in the sand. I had a sand box – nice and hot in the summer. And swimming. I used to go swimming – I learned to swim by the time I was five. Everybody swam on the lake anyway. And we would go down very often and have sort of the water treatment then.[45]

When Lina started school, she left behind her leg brace in favour of a pair of Oxford shoes. She walked with a slight limp, mostly corrected by the built-up sole of her left Oxford. Deeply grateful that she was not as immobilized by her polio as other children she knew were, Lina worked hard to keep up with her siblings and friends. For the most part, she was able to do so. "I had to walk [to school]," she remembered. "We had no busses at that time and I think we were at least a mile-and-a-half from school – and back again – so it was a good three-mile walk. I think that probably strengthened my leg quite a bit."[46]

Lina, like Lily, remembered her elementary school as a very significant provider of health services in the community. It was at school, she recalled, that she received medical and vision examinations and dental checkups. The school health nurse was regularly present and would issue notes to parents indicating any conditions that required follow-up treatment at home or by a doctor. "I can remember going when I was really young," Lina said. "Kelowna was a pretty progressive community ... we had all the up-to-date dentist and medical. It really was that kind of a town."[47] Lina believed that she was extremely fortunate to have grown up where she did during hard economic times. "I was a child in the Depression," she stated. "It didn't really affect the children as much as the parents, but I know being in the locality we were in – I think that makes the difference. Geography makes a big difference in the health of the child."[48]

CONCLUSIONS

The rhetoric of professional medical practitioners in the interwar period suggested they were solidly entrenched as the rightful arbitrators of the health and welfare of children. Doctors and nurses encouraged absolute compliance from parents in this regard, admonishing those who defied or ignored their authority.[49] Their confidence was earned in many respects: between the early 1930s and the beginning of the Second World War, death rates from contagious diseases that had been the scourge of childhood declined significantly (see Appendix 1: Causes of Infant Death in Canada, for five-year periods, 1921–50). The authority of medical practitioners and their approach to health and well-being, however, was never absolute nor even always the most important force that shaped health and illness in childhood. The experiences of Shirley, Lily, Jack, and Lina, like those of Florence, Marc, Alice, and Theresa decades earlier, testify to this. In the case of Shirley and Lily, challenges posed by the social context of the Great Depression had a very direct impact on familial and community responses to health needs. While Shirley's father was forced to move from one community to another in search of steady work, Lily recalled her family providing what little assistance they could to even less fortunate neighbours. Conversely, the relatively privileged family circumstances of both Jack and Lina meant that hardships associated with underemployed breadwinners or living on marginal agricultural land did not affect them.

The social consequences of attitudes towards class, gender, and race help us to account for these differences. As the experience of both Shirley and Lily suggest, First Nations peoples often occupied complex positions between traditional ways of life and those imposed by the dominant culture by the interwar period. As Robin Jarvis Brownlie has argued, paid work has a long history among First Nations, but securing it often meant dealing with racist attitudes and practices that often resulted in inadequate or underemployment. That First Nations peoples turned to traditional practices to sustain their families reflected this exclusion from paid work as much as it did on their desire to sustain their culture.[50] In the case of both Shirley and Lily, it seems far more likely that traditional cultural practices, such as hunting and trapping, were necessary given the inadequate opportunities presented, particularly to their fathers, in the white-dominated capitalist economy. Due primarily to his father's secure job in the tanning factory and her family's prosperous farm in the Okanagan Valley, Jack and Lina recalled far fewer bouts with economic hardship than did Shirley and Lily. As the daughter of Italian immigrants, Lina, much like Shirley and Lily, valued the close-knit Italian-Canadian Catholic community that surrounded her. Unlike Shirley and Lily, however, Lina's community seemed to supply primarily cultural enrichment rather than physical sustenance and refuge from an often overtly racist dominant culture.

All three women, however, recalled school as a place that occupied a formative position in their memories of growing up, albeit not always in a positive way. In this regard, Shirley's memories of racism and sexual harassment were the most painful and difficult. At the elementary level, she enjoyed school but this dissipated as she grew older. While Shirley recalled little of positive value from her later school years, Lily and Lina found great value in their school health curriculum. Unlike the memories of their contemporary, Jack, and those of Florence, Marc, Alice, and Theresa, who grew up decades earlier, health curriculum stood out for Lily and Lina as directly useful for protecting the well-being of their families.

A powerful theme linking all of the childhood memories explored in both chapters is the enduring importance of domestic doctoring and traditional medicine in family life. Existing parallel to the growing entrenchment of professional medical authority over the interwar decades, familial strategies of care retained their influence. Shirley, Lily, Jack, and Lina all recalled that mothers, or female relatives in particular, provided home remedies or used items purchased from travelling salesmen to alleviate pain and discomfort. Goose grease rubbed on backs, warmed oil poured in ears, or camphor smelling salts were prepared and administered in the hope of easing suffering. Lily recalled no less than four practitioners who dispensed variously successful treatments for her family. A favoured midwife/medicine woman provided much-needed relief to her mother and to her siblings, particularly when a new baby arrived. Conversely, an incompetent substitute midwife, along with a medicine man and a conventional male doctor, were far less skilled and successful in treating illness. Lastly, Lily's mother occasionally used home remedies for earaches or head lice, relying on tonics and creams purchased from travelling salesmen. Jack recalled that his mother acted as the "doctor" for his entire neighbourhood, dispensing not only effective treatments but also taking in children who were hungry. Lina's mother also relied on home remedies and purchased items from travelling salesman and provided massage therapy to help ease the symptoms of her daughter's polio.

A second powerful aspect that links the experiences of Shirley, Lily, Jack, and Lina with those of Florence, Marc, Alice, and Theresa are the deep and enduring connections between health concerns, familial circumstance, and social constraints. While Shirley, Lily, Jack, and Lina did not endure many of the typical childhood disease infections that plagued those born a few decades earlier, they nevertheless navigated significant challenges to their health and well-being. At the heart of these health challenges was the mitigating power of race, class, and gender. The further each family found themselves from the ability to share in, or mimic, white, middle-class, patriarchal values and mores, the more difficult it became to lay claim to good health and well-being.

4

Learning the Body: Schools, Curriculum, and Health

Over the turn of twentieth century, public schools were spaces where the dissemination of official information and values regarding the constitution of healthy living took place. Added to the public school curriculum in Canada in the late 1800s and often written by or with the help of medical professionals, health education advanced hegemonic conceptions of disease and disease prevention, sanitation and hygiene, and healthy and unhealthy bodies. In health classes, students learned about proper nutrition, the nature of disease-causing germs and bacteria, and the rules of public health and hygiene. They were measured, weighed, and inspected for dirt and lice, received vaccinations, eye examinations, and endured the extraction of teeth. More than simply presenting evolving rules of health, however, health education reflected a broader set of priorities on the part of medical professionals. A preoccupation in the curriculum with the detection, containment, and treatment of contagious diseases, gave way to a preventative approach to good health over the first decades of the twentieth century. Christian moral imperatives followed by newer emphases on health's role in "democratic living" as the century wore on helped justify the importance of health education to students and parents. Health in schools, in the estimation of some in the medical community, deserved to be "a subject which is inseparable from other subjects of the school curriculum, and that every teacher can help materially with this most important and vital part of the child's education."[1]

Schools are places that exert enormous power over the children that inhabit their halls and classrooms. As Keith Hoskins argues, "the child is controlled through the thorough organization of his time; the architecture of the school leaves him few zones of shade in which to hide; he is subject to the surveillance of teachers and prefects, and not infrequently that of his peers."[2] In this chapter, I demonstrate that the while the influence of schooling and school health curriculum in the lives of youngsters was impactful in a number of ways, it was never absolute nor uncontested. While the official curriculum was clear about children's roles and responsibilities in the cultivation of health and well-being over the first half of the century, memories of adults who recall their time in school make clear that youngsters and their families "talked back" to, and in the process modified, this influence in important ways.

Although school health curriculum has received limited attention from historians in the Canadian context, its roots reach back to the late 1800s.[3] Since education is administered provincially, decentralized provincial boards of education took the lead in establishing the official health curriculum in local settings. Textbooks, and in this case health education textbooks, represented a major component of the curriculum in Canada over the entire century.[4] In this chapter, I focus critical attention on conceptions of good health, disease prevention, and socially sanctioned morals and values that underpinned educative approaches to health and healthy children.[5] An analysis of textbooks alone, however, cannot tell us how they were taught in the classroom or how they influenced the mindset or behaviour of pupils.[6] Twentieth-century health teaching was never taken up consistently in all schools or by all educators, regardless of their importance in the context of a modernizing country.[7] This is clearly reflected in the range of experiences with health in school settings that emerge from oral history testimony. In the memories of some adults, learning to be healthy was a significant part of their education and made a positive difference in their lives. For others, formal lessons regarding health had little or no impact on home life. Still others recall quite negative associations between the expectations of healthful living promoted at school and their personal experiences. The exigencies of class, race, gender, and ability meant that some children incorporated lessons and expectations fostered in schools into their family life with ease while others found this difficult, if not impossible.

HEALTH CURRICULUM AT THE TURN OF THE CENTURY – INDIVIDUAL SALVATION AND THE RULES OF HEALTH

Compulsory school attendance laws in place in most provinces by the turn of the twentieth century established formal schooling as an integral part of childhood.[8] With its captive audience of children, schools were ideal settings for the dissemination of a range of hegemonic ideas, attitudes, and values. The promotion of hygiene – the science of sanitation – was an integral part of early professional efforts on the part of the medical establishment to control contagion and encourage "healthful living" amongst individuals, in neighbourhoods, and in broader communities. This theme was especially prominent in early health texts. In classrooms then, lessons devoted to health and hygiene supported other public health initiatives unfolding beyond school buildings.

Christian values, eugenics, and the supposed inevitability of unequal social relations informed scientific discussions surrounding the causes and prevention of poor health and disease. *Gage's Health Series for Intermediate Classes* (1896), authorized for use in middle schools in Manitoba and British Columbia, seized on the discourse of eugenics, heredity, and race suicide to dissuade young Canadians from indulging in alcohol:

> Probably no one ever suffered from all the diseases produced by alcohol, but all habitual drinkers sooner or later experience one or more of them. And their children are more likely to inherit stronger appetite for narcotics and a weaker will with which to control it ... The taking of a single glass of liquor, the eating of brandy sauce or wine jelly, may rouse this inherited desire, though its processor may not have discovered that the taint is in his blood; the appetite, becoming uncontrollable, may bring its owner to a drunkard's grave.[9]

Influenced by tenets of the Christian temperance movement, messages such as this called upon girls and boys to view abstinence from alcohol and tobacco as part of their healthful journey to adulthood.[10]

By 1910, authorized health texts began to concede that environmental factors – the state of cleanliness, health habits, and dwellings – helped determine individual health. Still significant, however, was heredity stock. As Dr A.P. Knight, professor of physiology at Queen's University in Kingston, Ontario and author of *The Ontario Public School Hygiene* (1910) wrote, "If you have followed the teachings of this book thus far, it must be clear to you now that our lives from birth until old age are shaped largely by two great influences: (1) by what we inherit from our parents, grandparents, or other ancestral relatives, and (2) by our environment, that is, by our surroundings."[11] Christian duty extended to the preservation and promotion of good health and it was up to individuals to decide whether or not to follow the teachings of experts. Early textbooks provided constant reminders that self-control and a cheerful acceptance of one's station in life were signs of robust health. This extended to the observance of traditional gender roles. In *The Essentials of Health – A Text-book on Anatomy, Physiology, and Hygiene* (1909), for example, children learned that

> what every boy and girl should aim to do is put his [*sic*] body under the control of his mind in matters relating to his own health. That is to say, he should so apply his understanding of the uses of the various organs of the human body and the effects of this or that treatment upon them, that he is able for the most part to avoid those things which will be harmful to his health and cultivate those things which will help to upbuild [*sic*] his physical and mental manhood ... Control of our own bodies, then, based upon a proper understanding of them, is the first step toward the attaining of true manhood or womanhood.[12]

In the social context of early twentieth-century Canada, girls would be expected to parlay healthful habits into motherhood and marriage while boys would prepare for public roles of breadwinning, leadership, and governance.[13]

Despite professional struggles over Canada's infant mortality rate and the seeming ubiquity of highly contagious childhood diseases, such as scarlet fever, mumps, measles, rubella, and tuberculosis, school children were admonished in health and hygiene textbooks to avoid contagious disease as another part of their Christian duty. Following on this theme, early textbooks placed the lion's share of blame for sickness and disease on the moral failings of the individual. Whether through ignorance, wickedness, or willful disobedience, poor health was presented as partly a matter of choice. In *How to be Healthy*, a 1911 textbook written by Manitoban doctor J. Halpenny and approved for use in elementary and middle schools in British Columbia, Alberta, Saskatchewan, Manitoba, Quebec, Nova Scotia, and Prince Edward Island, good health and vigour were unmistakably moral virtues reserved for those who chose to live "a sensible, normal life." By extension, those who struggled with poor health were cast with a pallor of immorality, bad choices, and weak wills. Students were instructed,

> when real difficulties come to us, let us meet them manfully, and win or lose, but never hold onto them or brood over them. This is the cause of much ill-health. Our right to be happy must not be interferred [sic] with by anything ... Once we begin to brood, our power to do difficult things and our course to face the trouble begins to fail. Thus we weaken ourselves.[14]

This discourse of moral weakness causing ill health took on heightened meanings in communities where racialized minorities, particularly First Nations peoples, were thought simply incapable by virtue of their "Indianness" of looking after their health.[15] Government officials at the time repeatedly blamed high rates of mortality amongst First Nations peoples not on the effects of colonization and the far-reaching disruption this caused, but to a far more damning cause: "Conditions peculiar to Indians."[16] The duty of Christian men and women to help safeguard the health of First Nations peoples legitimized colonization and inequality.[17] Such an organized program of domination proved tenacious. In the late 1940s, the Department of Indian Affairs continued to sponsor "Indian Baby Shows" in various regions around the country. The baby show reflected white anxiety regarding First Nation childrearing practices and marked a not-so-subtle attempt to convince First Nation parents to adopt the standards of the settler culture in this regard.[18]

Taking personal responsibility for good habits of health and hygiene was central in the early health curriculum textbooks. In an era before socialized medicine, professional health care was potentially expensive. For those in rural and remote communities, it could also be difficult to procure. Whether conceived as a Christian duty, an economic measure, or a matter of sheer survival, good health was a concern for families. Contagious diseases such as typhoid fever, measles, diphtheria, small pox, and whooping cough spread not only through individual families, but through entire communities quickly. Not surprisingly, health textbook curriculum encouraged students to follow particular health "rules" in order to avoid these diseases. Students were taught to surround themselves with fresh air; live in well-ventilated, clean, and spacious houses; dress in loose clothing; eat a variety of good foods; avoid tobacco, liquor, coffee, and tea; avoid excessive brain work; get plenty of sleep; indulge in moderate exercise; carefully train the bowels for regularity; and avoid contact with sick people.[19] Dr Knight, professor of physiology at Queen's University, reminded young readers "one thing is certain, that, if nations or individuals break the rules of health, they will be punished ... Nature will take no excuse for not knowing the rules."[20]

Given that such dictums about spacious accommodations, fresh fruit, and modern household conveniences were steeped in middle-class assumptions, many Canadian families simply did not or could not measure up. When contagion did make its way into communities, the prospect of being quarantined was feared, especially for working-class families. Jack McCrea, born in 1926 in Huntsville, Ontario and profiled in more depth in chapter 3, remembered that

> it was bad when you got measles or chicken pox or anything like that. They'd come over and put a big sign on your door – "Quarantined" – and nobody could come in and nobody could go out. And of course there was no phones in those days so you had to sort of depend on your neighbours to come and find out what you wanted or if they needed to get anything in town.[21]

Aware of the high stakes associated with quarantine, many families attempted to ward off contagion in ways that bore little resemblance to the "rules" laid out in school health curriculum. These efforts underscore the severity of contagions, the desire to escape their considerable wrath, and the tenacious belief in the power of domestic doctoring and familial folk remedies. Glenda Myers, born in Halifax in 1910, remembered wearing a camphor bag around her neck during the Spanish influenza outbreak of 1918. "After that [outbreak of 1918]," she concluded, "every winter almost we wore that little bag of camphor around our necks and we were healthy, we never had colds or anything."[22] Into the 1920s and well beyond, families continued to concoct their own folk remedies to check the spread of diseases. Kathryn Sutherland, who grew up in Toronto in the mid-1920s, remembered vividly her father painting the outside of her and her siblings' necks with iodine to prevent sore throats. "Now that was a strange one," she recalled, "and of course you hated that because you went back to school with this great big brown throat from the iodine."[23] She also remembered that if any of the children had whooping cough, her father would seek out a newly paved road. "Somebody told my father that if we breathed in the tar it would stop the cough, so I remember him trekking us all out there and we had to stand there and breathe in this tar ... and I don't know if it helped or not!"[24] Kyle Moss was born just after the Second World War and grew up in Peterborough, Ontario with his father and grandparents. His grandparents, according to him, "had some strange ideas about home medicine ... before we went to school [my grandmother] would take a teaspoon of raw ginger powder mixed with sugar and we'd have to eat that before we walked to school ... we'd be spitting half the way!"[25] Clearly, children did not always willingly accept homemade remedies.

Domestic doctoring complicated official school health curriculum that privileged "science" over what was dismissed as "superstition." Its importance in many of the oral histories explored in this book suggests it represented something far more central than simply superstition, quackery, or backwardness. It is telling that despite, or perhaps because of, clear evidence from adult memories about the centrality of folk health remedies in their childhood, textbooks took great pains to challenge these practices: "Great and unnecessary waste of life, health and vigour has resulted, and still results, from a neglect of scientific principles in regard to common things."[26]

Failure on the part of particularly working-class whites to heed the advice of established medical practitioners in the treatment of children was presented mostly as a matter of alterable ignorance. In a paper presented to the Canadian Nurses Association meetings in Toronto in 1918, Dr W. Chipman noted for example that unfortunate babies have to "fight from the very start ... Their mothers fought before them – fought in poverty, in ignorance and neglect – to give them birth; and so in poverty, ignorance, and neglect the child's life begins." Education for motherhood, however paternalistic, was seized upon as a hopeful antidote.[27] "Little Mothers Classes" aimed at teaching young girls to care for infants and were introduced in elementary schools in major cities like Toronto by the First World War.[28]

No amount of education, however, was thought to compensate for non-compliance with conventional health dictums amongst non-whites. George Duncan, medical officer of health for Victoria, British Columbia visited Japan and China in 1894 to "acquaint myself, as far as possible, with the health condition of the people from which at present British Columbia draws the bulk of her immigration." Without hesitation, he reported, "Chinese immigration is, from the point of view of health, the most dangerous element against which we have to contend."[29] Duncan was similarly certain of the dangers of new Indo-Canadian communities to the health standards of the province. East Indians were hardest hit by plagues of disease in their countries of origin, he noted, because "the natives live in unsanitary conditions ... in defiance in every way of the laws of hygiene ... the White population, comparatively speaking, obey sanitation laws."[30]

In non-white communities around the country, however, white medicine was not necessarily looked upon as effective or accessible. Like First Nation practices, the healing traditions of other non-white communities were certainly not reflected nor sanctioned in school health curriculum. Conceptions of "health" very much reflected the values, traditions, and habits of the dominant society. In an era when entrenched racism shaped the experience of Chinese immigrants who came to Canada, for example, cultivating familiar and effective methods for treating sickness was nevertheless often a matter of survival.[31] Sing Lim, born in Vancouver's Chinatown in 1915, and his family turned to neighbourhood herbalists for traditional ingredients for healing. In his autobiography, Lim recalled that Mr Kwong's remedies were "mostly vegetable ... hundreds of little drawers contained herbs: ginseng, seeds, dried buds and blossoms, taro roots, bark, and seaweed ... Other drawers held stranger things: dried insects, rhino skins, dried snakes, and lizards, and animal horns."[32] Even into the 1920s and 1930s, the prospect of utilizing white medicine, especially for First Nations peoples, was threatening and not undertaken lightly. In the case of children, the threat could take on even greater dimensions. When Minnie Aodla Freeman, an Inuit born in 1936 on Cape Horn Island in James Bay, developed impetigo as a young girl, the prospect of receiving care at the hands of white medical practitioners was a source of stress in her young mind. She recalled that "the word ... *naniasiutik* began to be mentioned often by my grandparents ... it can mean medicine, nurse, doctor, or a person who tends the sick ... to me, it meant horror, fear, and pain."[33]

FROM SELF TO COMMUNITY – HEALTH CURRICULUM BETWEEN THE WARS

By the end of the First World War, the Christian temperance discourse that blamed ill health on personal wickedness and inferior inheritance was tempered with a more nuanced set of health dictums in school curriculum. Health texts suggested that "now boys and girls should be happy, and they should not worry about sickness at all ... they should know that, even though they carefully carry out the rules of health, healthy bodies alone will not protect them from certain diseases."[34] This shift reflected changes in the state's role in protecting public health, the increasing entrenchment of conventional medicine as the arbitrator of healthy bodies, and the ideals of progressivism or the "new education" that were promoted in official educational discourse in North America beginning in the 1920s. Taking its cue largely from developments in child psychology, progressive educational philosophy sought to abandon what was understood as the worst of "formalist" or traditional pedagogy – strict classroom discipline and learning by memorization and drill – and replace it with child-centred learning, which focused on investigation, co-operation, and mutual respect.[35] In many schools, particularly in urban settings, school nurses became regular members of staff and were expected to act as partners with teachers in the presentation of health lessons.[36]

In this context, the "usefulness" of health curriculum became a more overt concern between the wars and suggests that at least some educators questioned its efficacy. The authors of the *Ontario Public School Health Book* (1925) surveyed teachers in the province to determine how to present health curriculum in a more engaging manner. They learned that "a suitable book in hygiene should be interesting to the pupils, free from technical terms, and contain only such physiology as is necessary; and that its aim should be to arouse a desire for proper living, to develop health habits, and to teach the pupils of our public schools some simple means for the prevention of disease."[37] This desire to make the subject of health more enjoyable to children and more readily applicable to their daily lives was reflected in a new crop of approved textbooks offered in the twenties and thirties. Teachers could now draw upon textbooks that used stories, poetry, and games to convey important lessons regarding cleanliness, prevention of infection, and "right living." In *The Safety Hill of Health* (1927), young students, encouraged to keep clean in a poem by the "Soap Fairy," were to "Use water and soap each day, to keep all dirt and germs away / Wash your body well with me, once or twice a week, you see."[38] Growing up in the 1930s in Penticton, British Columbia, Jenny Randall recalled that "we used to have a nurse come around ... and she had a little monkey puppet called Cocoa ... Miss Twitty was her name and she had a long blue uniform and she'd come and inspect all our nails just to see that they were clean."[39]

Serious structural problems in schools in Canada in the 1920s and 1930s stood in sharp contrast to these rather whimsical curricular approaches. Many schools across the country, particularly in rural settings, were notorious for lack of proper sanitation, washroom facilities, and even physical space enough for the number of students in attendance.[40] While urban schools could suffer from problems such as polluted water and poor lighting, rural schools were routinely reprimanded by school medical inspectors for various violations of public health standards.[41] School buildings could be very unhealthy places for children. Ingrid Cowlie attended a one-room schoolhouse in Wildwood, British Columbia in the early 1920s that housed six grades. While authorized health curriculum during this time warned teachers and children about the dangers of contagious diseases, Cowlie remembered that "the school had no electricity or running water. Water was brought in a bucket from my place ... it was kept in an enamel container with a tap. We all drank out of it from the same cup! Near the school were two outhouses, one for the boys and one for the girls."[42]

Cowlie's recollections were not unique. At the Cranberry Lake School in Malaspina, British Columbia, Kay Hodgson recalled that "we had outside toilets until 1933 – and no place to wash our hands!"[43] Not only was the physical plant of many schools inadequate, they were also remembered as places where disease and illness spread effortlessly from child to child. "We huddled in double-knit sweaters," recalled Robert Collins of his one-room schoolhouse in Saskatchewan in the mid-1920s, "feet like blocks of ice, noses always clogged, mouths stained black from Smith Brothers cough drops, hacking and sneezing in a cacophony of misery."[44]

The belief that successful health teaching relied only minimally on physiological knowledge characterized many textbooks used in primary grades. *Wide-Awake School*, published in 1931 and authorized for schools in Quebec and British Columbia, is a good example of this newer approach to health pedagogy that turned deliberately away from lessons grounded in physiology. Written in the form of a chapter book, *Wide-Awake School* tells the story of the school children of Drowsy Town and their efforts to improve their own health and that of their community. When they are challenged by the children in the neighbouring town to improve their school absentee record, miraculous transformations take place. Thanks to the efforts of the Drowsy Town children to stay healthy and thereby stay in school, the community itself is saved. The mayor in the book explains, we older people are trying to keep up with this health procession by cleaning up Drowsy Town. We now have clean streets. We are making a great fight to get rid of flies and mosquitos; a garbage man has been hired to collect all the garbage every Monday morning, and we have dug several ditches to drain the swamps. You have noticed that screens are on the windows and the town seems a different place from what it was a year ago. We owe much of this to you, because you were first to wake up.[45]

In the context of the "new education," economic hardship, and the distant rumblings of another war, health pedagogy thus became a vehicle for lessons in "waking up" civic responsibility and citizenship. Healthful habits were those that not only improved the individual's well being, they radiated outward and eventually strengthened entire communities.

Ultimately, the curricular goal of forming positive "health habits" was to foster happiness in oneself and service to others. In an effort to make the curriculum appealing, teachers of older children were encouraged to have their students fill out health scorecards and to compete amongst themselves and other classes for health points (see Appendix 3: My Health Record). The health scorecard promoted in *Health Essentials for Canadian Schools* (1938), part of the Canadian Hygiene Series, and prescribed by the minister of education for use in British Columbia, encouraged student participation in forming "health habits." The scorecard was divided in sections, such as posture: "books carried at arm's length, extended downward, and changed from one hand to the other, 1 point"; food: "no coffee, 2 points"; exercise: "one half hour (at least) of enjoyable outdoor recreational activity each day, 5 points"; and home environment: "quiet room for study, 2 points."[46]

Such efforts to make the curriculum appealing, however, could be lost on incompetent or uninspired teachers. In the memories of Jenny Randall and Mark Cameron, who also grew up in Penticton, British Columbia in the thirties, the subject of health in the higher grades tended to be relegated to the emerging subject of physical education. Jenny recalled, "our phys. ed. teacher taught health as well but she wasn't very good ... we had to *memorize* the health primer ... oh, you know it was so boring I just couldn't tell you what was in that book."[47]

"Once a week or rather every second week, we had a health session," Mark recalled of his physical education classes. "He [the teacher] would tell us the facts of life and how important it was to eat properly and all those simple little things and that was the nearest we came to doing anything about health."[48]

Despite such lost opportunities to use health curriculum for much grander goals, many interwar textbooks aimed at impressing upon young minds the concept of embodied democratic citizenship. The significantly titled *New Ways for Old* (1938) placed self-conscious emphasis on the connections between strong, healthy, able bodies, civic pride, and belonging to the nation:

> New beliefs about what education should do have made great changes in schools. Learning the three Rs was the chief activity of the old schools, but the aim of the new schools is learning to live ... "Learning to live," in a modern school, means that each boy and girl may grow strong and sturdy, in mind and body, and may become the best person possible for him [sic] to be, for his own sake, and for his home and community.[49]

Although health curriculum such as this prided itself on being innovative and cutting edge ("the aim of the new schools is learning to live"), several more traditional notions regarding healthy bodies endured. Cartesian dualism, the separation of body and mind, and self-control continued to influence how children and young adults were encouraged to think about their embodied selves.[50]

Behind admonishments regarding diet, study habits, and care of the body, textbooks gave credence to white and middle-class assumptions and anxieties regarding gender, race, and class at work in the interwar years. Textbooks aimed at a high school audience, for example, targeted girls' presumed interest in "beauty" as an opportunity to promote traditional attitudes towards health and gender. Authors discouraged young women from turning to the ever-expanding array of beauty products aimed at young consumers. Far from being healthful, they warned, some products were potentially lethal. "Some of the creams advertised for their miraculous powers contain lead," cautioned one author, "from which poisoning may arise ... No magic should be expected."[51] A 1938 textbook warned young women that the inexperienced use of makeup might have the effect of damaging wholesome reputations: "The best-looking people are usually the well-groomed and natural-looking ones. Scarlet cheeks and lips take away from the interest of one's eyes, and from the natural harmony of one's features. A natural glow is more attractive than the most artful make-up."[52] Securing a "natural glow" was presumed to be an important goal for young girls. All "natural glows," however, were not equally acceptable. The appearance of acne, a condition that plagued youngsters of both sexes, is discussed solely as a failure to adhere to winning health habits. Harkening back to the notion that bad choices resulted in ill health, textbooks continued to blame the weak individual for their condition. Those youngsters unfortunate enough to suffer from acne, despite efforts to deal with it, would have learned that "skin disturbances are common especially among young people who do not choose a well-balanced diet, or those who neglect sleep, rest, or outdoor exercise, or their habits of personal cleanliness."[53]

Interwar health textbooks promoted home settings and eating habits associated with urban Anglo-Celtic, middle-class traditions as the healthiest and therefore most socially acceptable. Foods such as potatoes, beans, spinach, onions, string beans, squash, cauliflower, parsnips, turnips, daily rations of lean meat, eggs, and whole-grain breads, are singled out and promoted as healthy fare.[54] In *Healthy Citizenship* (1935), the authors offered detailed descriptions of "good housing," that included a free-standing home, a garden plot, surrounding yard, lots of sunlight and fresh air, and a sleeping porch.[55] Children would also learn that particular furnishings, including newer lightweight carpets and draperies, domestic technology such as vacuum cleaners, and washing with ample amounts of hot water, characterized the healthy home. Families in more crowded circumstances, in apartment complexes, or perhaps in multi-family dwellings, without modern conveniences, and who ate foods not sanctioned in health curriculum would not find themselves reflected in state-sanctioned notions of good health.

It is important to consider, therefore, the implications of such curriculum goals for children and families judged outside the boundaries of white, middle-class society. The experiences of Shirley and Lily highlighted in the previous chapter, for example, make clear that racist attitudes towards First Nation peoples exacerbated challenges to good health and, at worse, directly threatened good health. For First Nation children confined to various residential schools across the country, healthy living was not typically a priority in their education. Quite the contrary, they came to represent places where many children became extremely ill and/or died.[56] Minnie Aodla Freeman recalled of her time at St Thomas Anglican School in Moose Factory in the 1940s, "their bannock was terrible ... I forced it all down ... a few times I could force myself ... out it would come with the force of a strong leak in a canoe, all over the floor ... I would be put to bed, my forehead would be felt and my temperature taken. That's when I felt most lonely, in this great big bedroom with two hundred beds in it."[57] Through health education in residential schools, as Mary-Ellen Kelm has shown, "children were taught to hate the food their mothers cooked and reject their standards of cleanliness ... school officials told students that cultural alienation was to be welcomed as the first step towards healthful living and long life."[58] Through health curriculum, food and space became not only racialized and classed, but acted as indices of membership within the bounds of Canadian citizenship.[59]

Whether or not students took health lessons to heart, and what was at stake for them if they adhered to or neglected them was a complex and varied proposition. Despite the largely negative experience of residential school for Minnie Aodla Freeman, for example, the fact that health and hygiene lessons were offered in classes made a significant difference to her family at least on one important occasion. When her father was struck with pneumonia she was able to put what she had learned about health to good use by making a mustard plaster to ease his suffering. She credits this plaster with helping her father recover from his terrible illness.[60] Marion Gallagher attended school in Victoria, British Columbia in the 1930s and recalled "all our belongings had to be labelled and a fresh, clean, ironed cotton handkerchief brought to class every day!"[61] Robert

Collins' experience was, however, very much the opposite. According to him, the teacher rarely discussed health. When it was brought up, the subject matter was distinctly forgettable. "We raised our fingernails for inspection," Collins remembered, "and lied about whether we had brushed our teeth, drunk eight glasses of water, and slept for eight hours ... so much for the subject known as health."[62] When asked if she recalled being examined by a school nurse, Eileen Davies, who grew up in Barrie, Ontario in the 1940s, said, "Not that I remember. I think I can remember a nurse coming to the school – what was it for – to talk about hygiene, I think. Maybe it was for shots. I don't recall. Whatever it was, it didn't make a big impression anyway."[63] Similarly, Frank Johnson who attended a First Nation band school in the British Columbia interior in the 1950s stated, "I remember rolling this big barrel of skimmed milk and carrying boxes of some kind of crackers or pilot biscuits or something home that the school provided ... so that was the school's nutrition program."[64] Some informants, however, remembered considerable social shame accompanied their family's nonconformity to official teaching about healthy habits. Although she grew up learning in health classes that youngsters were to bathe daily, Doris MacKenzie, raised in Montreal during the 1940s, listened as her mother felt compelled to lie to doctors about her family members' less acceptable habit of bathing only weekly.[65]

CONCLUSIONS

Health textbook curriculum was designed to influence how school children not only thought about and cared for their bodies, but how these practices supported social values promoted by the dominant culture. Christian tenets of self-control, cleanliness, and adherence to "rules" appropriate to the respectable classes were promoted in health curriculum early in the century. After the end of the First World War and in the midst of considerable social change, new themes emerged. Spurred on by changing scientific understandings of germ theory and disease prevention, as well as new educational philosophies that privileged progressive approaches to learning, health curriculum aimed to persuade children to foster healthy lives as a conduit to strong national identity and democratic citizenship. On and through children's bodies, social acceptability, civilizing and colonizing techniques, interests of the state, and so-called "good health" were written, operationalized, and vied for space.

When this expert-driven discourse is complemented with the memories of adults from diverse backgrounds who grew up in Canada over the period examined, a richer understanding of how these discursive constructions were lived within families comes to the forefront. The lived memories of adults who grew up in different communities in Canada suggest that the inculcation of particular kinds of health lessons did not go uncontested nor were they simply received and integrated into childhood experience in uncomplicated ways. Health curriculum could indeed make a difference in the way some children learned about their bodies, but it was not simply an expert-imposed process. What was at stake in terms of cultural safety varied considerably depending on where one was positioned in the hierarchical social ladder that characterized Canada over the twentieth century. The way curriculum and medical experts, teachers, and parents thought about and treated children's bodies reproduced and challenged relations of power. Through the body, children learned and took up their various places in the hierarchal world of their families and communities.

5

Treated Bodies: Hospitalization

In the early months of 1914, siblings Gina and Thomas Sharon were discharged from Toronto's Hospital for Sick Children[1] with only "slight improvements" to their congenital syphilis.[2] Gina was three-and-a-half years old. Her brother was two. Brought to the hospital by their father, the children stayed for three months. The records do not reveal why their father brought them to the hospital when he did, whether he knew of their condition beforehand, or how the children fared during and after their long hospitalization. While the record is silent on precisely why the siblings were admitted when they were, congenital syphilis in children who survive past birth invites a range of serious conditions, including bone pain, joint swelling, blindness, and deafness.

In the spring of that same year, nine year-old Paula Friedman was admitted to HSC after she hemorrhaged following the extraction of a tooth. In their brief case notes, the doctors speculated that Paula suffered from hemophilia. Her condition quickly improved, however, and she was discharged after only three days on the ward.

When eight-year-old Moira Tyndell was admitted to the hospital on 25 February 1914, she had been suffering from coughing, headaches, vomiting, fever, and distressed and rapid breathing the previous four days. Staff recorded that she was an "only child" and speculated about her diagnosis. They noted that Moira might well be suffering from advanced pneumonia, a congenital heart defect, or rheumatic fever. By March, her record indicated that she was gradually improving: "Breathing is not so distressed and child is coughing less." This, unfortunately, did not last. At 8:00 a.m. on 13 April 1914, after another month of battling considerable respiratory distress, Moira died.

Between March and May of 1914, three unrelated boys ranging in age from one month to one year also died in hospital from what Dr Alan Brown, their young physician, labelled "fermentative diarrhea." Such cases motivated Brown to devote much of his professional career to improving the feeding habits of babies and young children. In 1930, along with his colleagues Fred Tisdall and Theo Drake, Brown invented the first ready-to-use baby cereal, Pablum.[3] Enriched with vitamin D and other minerals, Pablum marked a groundbreaking advancement in nutritional science.[4]

Mary Michaels was admitted to the hospital at the end of January of 1915 with a diagnosis of masturbation due to "moral degeneracy." A clitoridectomy was preformed five days later and after a month in hospital she was declared "cured" and discharged. Mary was nine years old. Chester Bullen was seven years old when he was admitted on 11 May 1916. He remained in hospital for three months. With few details, his chart indicated that he suffered bullet wounds to both hands and his right arm. He "improved," however, and was eventually sent home.[5]

Attention to the health needs of the young resulted in specialized health curriculum in schools, specialized sites in the form of children's hospitals, such as Toronto's HSC, and specialized doctors in the form of pediatricians and specialists in adolescent medicine over the late nineteenth and early twentieth centuries in North America.[6] The profiles that open this chapter, randomly chosen from early twentieth-century patient records at HSC, capture a small fraction of the daily drama that unfolded there over the century. They provide only fleeting impressions of the children whose illnesses or conditions, in an era before publicly funded health services, were judged serious enough to warrant hospitalization.[7] We learn nothing about how the children themselves felt about their hospitalization or their treatment at the hands of hospital staff. Nevertheless, the patient records hint at the range and severity of challenges to the health and well-being of children living in or traveling to Canada's largest city in the early years of the twentieth century.

The oral histories gathered for this book provide new and different perspectives on the provision of both formal and informal, or familial health services for young children in the context of Canada. As I explored in the previous chapter, school health curriculum contributed to a particular construction of the "healthy child" that embedded white, middle-class values and sensibilities into the very heart of what it meant to be healthy. For their part, children and their families variously reproduced, ignored, and challenged this expert-driven curriculum, imbuing it with meanings that often ran contrary to the intended message.

Hospitals mark another pre-eminent location where the formal provision of health services also saw complex interactions among staff, parents, and child patients. While a number of studies have traced the history of the development of hospitals, hospital services, and their connection to health policy, the perspectives of child patients on this history have been largely absent.[8] Denyse Baillargeon's study of leisure and learning inside Sainte-Justine Hospital in Montreal explores efforts to include play therapy, scholastic advancement, and moral uplift into activities aimed at young patients. While Baillargeon does not engage the perspectives of the young, her work is nonetheless valuable for our understanding of attempts to support the well-being of hospitalized children.[9] With an interpretive emphasis on hospital architecture, Annmarie Adams' engaging study charts the changing priorities in hospital design in the twentieth century and the role of (particularly middle-class) patients in driving this change. The provision of children's wards and wings is illustrated by the example of the evolution of Montreal's Royal Victoria Hospital and demonstrates the modern hospital's receptivity to the health needs of specific patient populations.[10]

Drawing primarily on oral histories, patient records from the HSC, and, to a lesser degree, the writings of medical professionals over the early to mid-decades of the twentieth century, I explore and contextualize in this chapter memories of women and men who spent time in hospital during their childhood. Here, I build upon and complement the memories of visiting or staying in hospitals in the experiences of Florence, Marc, Alice, and Theresa explored in detail in chapter 2. In this chapter, memories of hospitalization in childhood continue to be revelatory in a number of important ways. They provide a perspective largely absent from the Canadian context: how children experienced the institutional setting of the hospital, away from the familiarity and comfort of their families, often for long periods of time, and with the added stress of illness or injury. This perspective, I argue, reminds us that a complex dynamic not simply dictated and driven by adult agendas shaped attitudes towards the young and the experience of being young. The institutional setting of the hospital, the priorities and capabilities of hospital staff, attitudes towards children, and the experiences of children themselves each contributed a layer of complexity.

HOSPITALIZATION, PROFESSIONALS, AND THE PROVISION OF CHILD-CENTRED CARE

In the early decades of the twentieth century, many children visited the hospital for treatment. This was the case for acute and emergency treatment, as well as for non-emergency appointments with doctors. An analysis of pediatric admissions to Kingston General Hospital between 1889 and 1909 sheds light on the reasons for children's hospitalization in one mid-sized Canadian city at the turn of the twentieth century.[11] In keeping with broader trends across the country in this early period, contagious diseases such as tuberculosis, measles, diphtheria, scarlet fever, and typhoid fever accounted for the largest percentage of admissions (28.5 per cent) amongst children aged fourteen and under.[12] Tonsil and adenoids (17 per cent); organ infections, such as bronchitis or mastoiditis (14.7 per cent); male circumcisions (12 per cent); conditions related to infections, such as nephritis (8.8 per cent); surgical cases (7.8 per cent); accidents and injuries (5.8 per cent); treatment of congenital conditions, such as cleft palate (1.7 per cent); conditions caused by nutritional deficiencies (1.1 per cent); and other conditions (2.6 per cent), including skin irritations, and in the case of one girl, pregnancy, made up the remaining reasons for admissions.[13]

In remote towns and villages around the country, small, modest hospitals often fulfilled the additional function of extended-term residence for patients. This was true of adults as well as children.

The R.W. Large Memorial Hospital on the Heiltshuk Indian reserve in Bella Bella, British Columbia stands as one example. Patients, including children, typically travelled far distances to receive treatment at the hospital and often stayed for long periods of time. Florence Moffatt, a nurse at the hospital, recalled a typical patient experience in the 1940s: "Beatrice was a young Indian girl who had been at the hospital for more than two years recovering from tuberculosis ... a steamer would arrive to transport her back home to Kitamaat. Such was the way of life in those days, on an island where boats were the only mode of transportation."[14]

In larger urban centres, and increasingly over the twentieth century, children's experience with hospitalization began at birth. As Cynthia Comacchio and Wendy Mitchinson have shown, a central component of the medicalization of childbirth involved hospitalization.[15] Hospital birth, touted as the "modern" alternative to home birth, was promoted as an important safeguard against maternal and infant mortality, and was seen to be in keeping with faith in medical science that permeated the early twentieth century. Education for "scientific motherhood" began in hospital shortly after the child was born and continued through the work of neighbourhood well-baby or child hygiene clinic visits.[16] Over the course of the twentieth century, hospitals evolved as sites of medical treatment – emergency and outpatient – to include research and experimentation, and the provision of broader social welfare services.[17]

Hospital procedures regarding child patients varied considerably across context and time period. One exception to this variation, however, involved patient visitations. In the early decades of the twentieth century it was common for children's hospitals or children's wards to severely curtail patient visitations. Such restrictions rested on a number of assumptions: first, that children would become accustomed to hospitalization more readily if family visits were infrequent and short, and second, such restrictions would curtail the spread of infections. While it was an early leader in child-centred hospital care in other domains, Sainte-Justine Hospital in Montreal, as Denyse Baillargeon has shown, restricted visiting hours.[18] For much of the mid-1930s, standard practice at HSC also saw visitation for public ward patients limited to one hour on Sunday afternoons.

Parents viewed their hospitalized infants through a window or sat beside their older children's hospital bed. Rarely did parents have an opportunity to interact with medical staff during these visits. As Judith Young describes in her work on the HSC: "In the admitting department the child was separated from the parent, examined, and sent to the ward ... [W. Hawk, a pediatric resident at HSC: in 1935] likened the system to that of a 'Chinese laundry' where packages were left and then picked up by the parent when treatment was complete."[19] Despite efforts by nursing staff and junior physicians to expand visiting hours, and research showing the psychological toll that separations took, daily visiting on the public wards was not introduced at HSC until 1961, and even later at Sainte-Justine. Even when extensions were granted, visitation of patients was still confined to three hours in the afternoon. In 1965, all-day visiting from 11:00 a.m. until 8:00 p.m. was introduced at HSC.[20]

A 1946 editorial in *Maclean's* magazine by Dr W.W. Bauer, director of the Bureau of Health Education for the American Medical Association, suggested that professionals increasingly recognized, and grappled with, the possible psychological and emotional damage that hospitalization could mean for children. Drawing on the popularity of psychological discourse, Bauer warned of a constellation of mental health issues that could result from long-term hospitalization of the young:

> It's a severe emotional strain to remain abed, isolated from playmates and from normal living, for many months. A year is longer in childhood than in later life. It not only (seems) longer – it is longer, in development, growth, and significance. In that time a child may fall so far behind his normal companions that he never catches up; out of this may grow a serious sense of failure and frustration. Constant attention may make him neurotic. The instinct to dominate, to use the natural anxiety of the parents as a lever to secure attention, may become overdeveloped. Or he may so abhor any semblance to get him, later on, to take proper care of himself.[21]

The assumed threat to normalcy posed by an interrupted childhood helped motivate some practitioners to pay close attention to the emotional needs of hospitalized children. Like the example of patient visitation, however, the inclusion of play greatly varied according to context and time. The Children's Memorial Hospital of Montreal, for example, developed a new branch of its nursing service, Recreational Therapy, in the mid-1930s. Introducing the branch to the readership of *The Canadian Nurse* in 1937, Alice Buckhardt explained that its "chief function is to educate the nursing staff to the use of play as a means of facilitating nursing procedure and to create, through play with the children, the normal environment to which every child is entitled."[22] The use of structured play, Buckhardt reported, had several important strengths. First, as is suggested above, play therapy helped nurses carry out their tasks more efficiently and, with a happy, co-operative patient, more effectively. Play therapy also, according to Buckhardt, brought something familiar to the child in the otherwise "strange smelling and foreboding environment" of the hospital. "In this hospital," she pronounced, "play therapy has proven itself an invaluable aid in solving many problems and we have found play to be the best medium through which to gain whole-hearted cooperation."[23] In her 1955 description of the pre- and post-operative care of a young patient, Winnipeg nurse Esme Baker suggested that play was an important way to maintain "home associations." Before her operation, "Lucy was encouraged to join in play with other little girls her age. Stories were read and enjoyed."[24] Albeit it with important adjustments, play was also considered an important component of post-operative care for Lucy. "She was assisted to sit up the third day post-operatively as her chest sounded congested and a loose, harsh cough developed ... Play had to be within her strength, limited post-operatively to books, dolls, conversation with nurses and other children ... This kept up her home association."[25]

Hospitalized in 1956 in Ottawa after breaking his arm, William Sweeney remembered that the hospital was "a spooky place for an eight-year-old kid." Surrounded by other children in the large public ward, however, William remembered that play provided a welcome distraction. While he did not recall structured programs of play offered by the nursing staff, children certainly gravitated towards one another. "It was kids in wheelchairs and kids with broken arms and sort of a common room," he remembered, "with a television, black and white and there was nothing on it, but we found a way to have fun, we sort of played."[26]

At HSC, recommendations for the introduction not only of open visiting, but of recreation programs and "psychosocial training of nurses and physicians," were not formally addressed until the late 1960s. Suggesting that play therapy was not a regular aspect of care for children in all hospitals, Françoise Miller Ouellet's 1960 article encouraged colleagues to consider introducing it into their practice:

> As a first step in providing a recreation program, there should be a special area set aside for this purpose to give the child a change of scene, to take him out of an environment of illness and provide an opportunity for social contact with other boys and girls. It would be even more desirable to have two or three rooms large enough so that children who are up and about or who can get around on crutches, etc. may be able to move freely. The nurse should see to it that the arrangement of the department encourages this. It should even be possible to bring patients in their beds so that bedridden children can participate as well.[27]

Miller Ouellet's advice made clear that a major aim of recreational programming involved taking patients out of "an environment of illness" represented by the hospital itself. The ideal setting, as Miller Ouellet advised, involved large dedicated spaces, away from the wards, where children with a range of mobilities could "move freely," interact with other children, and perhaps forget, if only temporarily, that they were not at home, surrounded by the familiar and familial. Her advice, directed as it was specifically to nurses, also suggest that responsibilities in this regard fell primarily on their shoulders.

THE CASE OF MICHAEL LONDELL[28]

The patient record of Michael Londell, only five months old when he was first admitted to the HSC on 2 October 1930, provides a window onto another set of priorities for those responsible for hospitalized children. Constructed from the vantage point of hospital staff,

Michael's record reveals how closely nurses and doctors worked with social services, including social workers, and how expectations regarding the "good child" and the "good family" informed professional judgements of Michael's health status. Largely absent from Michael's record, however, are clues as to whether therapeutic services, such as recreational play therapy or other attempts to foster "home associations" were part of his experience.

Michael was admitted to the HSC in early October 1930 with a diagnosis of nasopharyngitis (inflammation of the nasal passages and the upper part of the pharynx) and "infectious diarrhea." A physical examination revealed that he was a "well developed and nourished child."[29] After a two-month stay in hospital, Michael was discharged. In his fifth year, on 27 January 1935, Michael was again admitted to the hospital. This would mark the beginning of a six-month stay. His list of ailments was significant: "acute rheumatic fever, possible chorea?, thymus enlarged, flat feet and knocked kneed, appendectomy." Hospital staff also noted his previous admittance to the HSC for "intestinal intoxication" and a concussion suffered when he was three years old. His record reveals a steady decline in his health and an increasing level of professional intervention towards the end of the 1930s and into the 1940s:

> This child has been repeatedly in hospital ... since 5 years of age has been coming in for bouts of rheumatic fever – has been in once or twice every winter since." The last time was approximately one year ago, December 1939, when he was in hospital 2-3 months. Since that admission, he has had repeated attacks of pain in calves, knees, and shoulders ... influenza, cough, head cold, fever, attends cardiac clinic.

Patient information gathered for Michael's transfer to the cardiac clinic suggest that professional staff believed that his family circumstances held the key to his poor health. Michael was one of five children that included four boys, aged eighteen (had joined the army), sixteen, thirteen, nine (Michael), and one girl, aged fourteen. His parents were listed as separated. His mother, a housewife, was recorded as "not well – nervous – and attends outpatient clinic department at Women's College Hospital," while his father was listed as "working at Westinghouse." The family's monthly income of seventy-nine dollars meant that while they were not poor, they were far from comfortably middle class. Home visits judged the family house to sit on good residential land but had no play facilities nearby, had crowded living space, was inadequately heated (bad furnace), poorly ventilated, and was "very dirty and disorderly." A number of dietary inadequacies were noted. Even though the family used two quarts of milk a day, Michael drank none. It was noted that he did not eat meat daily, had two servings of vegetables a day, no juice, but plenty of bread and grains. His school was located three blocks from his home and his classroom was on the second floor. The record noted that Michael climbed the two flights of stairs three or four times per day in order to get to his classroom.

The hospital staff, in conjunction with social services, tried to address and alleviate conditions that were interpreted as challenging to Michael and his family. First, steps were taken to limit the amount of climbing that Michael had to endure to reach his classroom. "Arrangements have been made from year to year," the record stated, "that the boy be placed in a grade on the ground floor." Coping with his mother's inadequate homemaking skills proved to be more difficult, however. "Much work has been done on this home through the public health nurse and visiting home mothers – with result that Mrs Londell is a very poor housekeeper, well-known to neighbourhood workers' associations."

Michael's final admission to the hospital occurred on 27 December 1944 at the age of fourteen. He was found to have a congenital malfunction of the heart, as well as hypertension. Rounding out his diagnoses was his "behaviour problem." This time, he would spend a year at the HSC. Staff recorded that he had suffered "recurring problems with rheumatic fever, severe nosebleeds that lasted three or four weeks, teacher noticed a marked mental dullness and he complains of dizziness and 'tightness' in the head – very apathetic and mopes a great deal." Upon his discharge on 7 January 1945, the patient record stated:

> Discharged today with instructions to remain in bed 14 hours out of 24 – attend morning school – start on thyroid gr./5 5 each

morning and return to cardiac clinic in two weeks. He was seen by Dr Boyer this morning who felt that this was an environmental rather than a neurological problem. A social worker calls at this home regularly.

Michael's record at the HSC provokes as many questions as it provides clear answers. While he and, by extension, his family faced a number of health challenges, there are limited indications of his reaction to his hospital encounters. How, for example, did Michael feel about his year-long hospitalization? Did he balk at the decision to move from his original classroom to one on the first floor of his school or did this please him? Did family and friends make regular visits? How did he spend his time? Was he bored, sad, angry, happy? How are we to interpret his "behavioural problem"? Did he have opportunities for play and recreation with other children? The record indicates hospital staff made considerable efforts to improve Michael's health, particularly scrutinizing his family life. These efforts also reveal, however, that his family was brought under increasing social surveillance, culminating in the clear suggestion that their, and particularly his mother's, inability to mimic the standards of middle-class domesticity contributed significantly to Michael's ill health. Indeed, a discourse of shame and blame tend to characterize health professionals' approach to the "problem" of Michael's mother. Michael's behaviour, too, was ultimately singled out as problematic by professionals who duly noted and psychologized his inability to comply as patient and child. That illness, physical discomfort, and long separations from family could provoke difficult behaviour was never suggested as a possible explanation by professionals. The patient record, in other words, tells us more about the assumptions and attitudes of hospital staff and the context of increasing professional surveillance in the 1930s and 1940s than it does about Michael and his family.

MEMORIES OF HOSPITALIZATION

Childhood memories of stays in hospital offer a deeper engagement with the kinds of professional narratives exemplified in the patient record of Michael Londell. They also provide clear evidence of some of the consequences and reactions that professional attitudes towards and treatment of small bodies had for children and their families. Adults remembered their childhood experiences with hospitalization along a spectrum from very positive to very negative. Marc Trapier, profiled in more detail in chapter 2, greatly valued his time in a quarantine hospital at the age of fourteen since it meant a respite from work. Andrea Knott, who grew up in Stoughton, Saskatchewan in the 1920s, recalled with great fondness her stay in the hospital for a tonsillectomy. "It was wonderful," she said. "It was just different, another experience." Part of the appeal rested in the fact that Andrea met another girl her age on her ward and made a lifelong friend. "She and I went to school together and we still correspond at Christmas."[30] When her appendix ruptured at the age of nine, Jenny Randall from Penticton, British Columbia spent ten days in hospital. "Well, I had surgery and a drainage tube and I was only nine but I quite enjoyed it up there; I made friends with the nurses and got pampered a little bit," she recalled. "I remember the nurses sneaking chocolates and things under my pillow."[31]

For other children the culture of hospitalization and nursing practice in the early decades of the twentieth century made their experience more difficult. Long separation from family members, so common a practice in many hospitals in aid of encouraging the child to adjust to hospital routines, limit the spread of infection, and in keeping with many families who could not afford the loss of work associated with hospital visits, was nevertheless traumatic from the point of view of many children. Monica Welsh, hospitalized at the age of twelve for pneumonia in the early 1940s, for example, associated her hospital experience with extreme loneliness:

[It was] scary to be away from home and being really, really, sick. [*Did you have family members staying with you at the hospital or were you staying by yourself?*] No! Absolutely and totally alone, not mom or dad or anybody ... Mom and dad milked cows and they were busy, and they had to be home throughout the day to milk cows and there wasn't anybody.[32]

Both Irena Friedman, born in rural New Brunswick in 1945, and Donald Traster, born in 1950 in Brockville, Ontario, shared Monica's experience of loneliness and fear. Their memories of hospitalization for tonsillectomy and appendectomy respectively, particularly in terms of feelings of isolation, loneliness, and uncertainty, are strikingly similar. Irena recalled being prepared for her surgery:

> I saw them come in the morning and put me in my little white gown, and I will never forget that – put me in a bed and didn't have, like, valiums or whatever they calm you down with – whatever they give to kids – and they just rolled me into a room with big, big bright lights – they were big, like flood lights. And um, they put this thing on my face, this huge mask. And I remember the smell of ether, and to this day I cannot stand the smell of ether.[33]

Traumatic memories of being anesthetized are also present in Donald's recollections:

> I can remember going into the operating room ... the bright lights and the doctors and nurses with their masks on. One vivid memory is how much the ether stung my face. And they put, like, these rubber things down and around my nose first and they administered the ether. But I can remember thinking how much it was burning.[34]

The feelings of vulnerability and uncertainty articulated by Irena and Donald echo in Trisha Price's experiences while in hospital. Born in 1948 and raised just outside of Kelowna, British Columbia, she recalled: "I did not enjoy being isolated in all this white. White walls with nurses around me, with strangers, and my throat hurt and I did not like going to this place where I was under someone else's authority ... there was one [nurse] who was just nasty ... and the others were just very business-like – they certainly didn't fuss over me."[35]

Vulnerability and loss of control were key themes in Gladys Rupert's memories of hospitalization as well. Gladys grew up with her younger brother in a tourist lodge located between Bracebridge and Huntsville in northern Ontario in the 1950s. Gladys's mother, a single parent, worked at the lodge as part of the cooking and cleaning staff. At the age of sixteen, Gladys had tonsillectomy surgery.

Afterwards, however, she developed an infection and began to hemorrhage. Gladys was eventually rushed to the hospital. Adding to the intensity of the experience was the fact that she had recently begun to menstruate:

> Anyway they took me into emergency and they were trying to take my clothes off and I was valiantly trying to keep my pants on because I had my period. And I couldn't talk. I was just gurgling. And they kept trying to pull my pants off and you know I didn't know why they couldn't see that I had a sanitary napkin on. Finally, Dr A just gave me a shot and that knocked me out and that was the end of the fight.[36]

When asked if she remembered any other details of her ten-day stay in the hospital, Gladys recalled that her bed was in a hall outside the maternity ward "because they had no room for me." She was not the only youngster for whom surrender of control was traumatic:

> There was this one little boy, they took his tonsils out and in those days they would tell the parents not to come near because it would make things worse if they came and left, so he screamed for two days straight. [A doctor] would come and give him a shot and knock him out ... he was in the hall, too.[37]

Based on assumptions regarding children's capacity to understand and cope with their health challenges, information about their condition or their treatment was often withheld from them or only briefly explained. Donald Traster recalled that his treatment was explained to him only "vaguely ... it was explained in very childlike terms like 'we're just going to take you in this room and you're going to fall asleep and when you wake up, you'll be all better ... you'll be a little sore.'"[38] While the experience of being "acted upon" was common for hospitalized children, evidence from oral histories suggests that youngsters also acted and re-acted on their own behalf and in their own interests with varying degrees of effectiveness. The screaming boy in Gladys's memories serves as one example. At one point, Donald refused to let the nurses bathe him during his hospitalization in Brockville: "I can remember the nurses wanting to bathe me and I wouldn't let them do it, and I would do it myself." He developed a severe case of shingles:

> The shingles had gone all the way around my back and were at my sides when they discovered it. And the reason it took so long to discover it is because I would do my own bathing and that kind of thing. And it was actually one of the doctors that discovered it first and I can remember him being very upset and yelling almost. He was screaming at the nurses and asking why they hadn't picked this up beforehand.[39]

Eileen Davies, born in 1943 outside of Barrie, Ontario, spent time in hospital for the removal of her tonsils and adenoids when she was five years old. She wanted very much to please and impress her doctor, Dr Taylor, and remembers vowing to "be good – because I liked him, you know, and I didn't want to disappoint him." Her postoperative discomfort, however, made this vow difficult to keep:

> After I came out of the anesthetic and, you know, I had a sore throat and I was feeling miserable and then I was told that I had to stay there for a couple of days, and I was ... [pause] ... apparently, I was a real brat. I wanted to go home, and I didn't want to be there, you know, they were holding me hostage. And I was not co-operative at all. My mother says that she remembers coming to visit me in the hospital and being greeted at the entrance of the ward with: "Are you Eileen's mother?" And when she said "yes," the reply was, "oh, good."[40]

Although Eileen recalls her bad behaviour with some regret, it also represented a form of knee-high agency. She acted out and, in the process, made it clear that she would not simply suppress her physical and emotional discomfort in the name of being a "good patient."

CONCLUSIONS

While considerable shifts in the way staff, particularly nurses, treated and understood hospitalized children were advocated in the professional discourse, these were neither straightforward nor universally implemented. Early advocates of recreational programming understood and promoted a correlation between children's sense of security and familiarity and their compliance with treatment protocols. Happy and secure children made good patients. This theme was picked up in the post-war period and was increasingly wedded with psychological reasoning. Failure to pay attention to the needs of children hospitalized for extended periods of time, risked producing neurotic, fearful, and incompetent citizens. Underneath the calls for nursing staff to "play while you nurse" was the sometimes tacit, sometimes explicit recognition that children had a unique set of needs that set them apart from adult patients.

Adult memories suggest that the uneven dynamics of power that characterize relations between children and adults had particularly challenging consequences in the context of hospitalization. That children were expected to accept the authority of adults gave medical professionals, already bestowed with considerable social power, additional control over their experiences. Not surprisingly, a heightened sense of powerlessness marked an important theme in the oral histories and was the result of the decisions and actions of medical professionals. Children's sense of powerlessness was largely the result of the actions and priorities of adults: the physical space of the hospital with its distinctly institutional character, bright lights, and unfamiliar, strong smells; absence of family, often made worse by strict limits on visitations; discomfort and fear associated with feeling ill or experiencing pain; boredom and sometimes harsh or indifferent treatment at the hands of staff. While some adults testified that they were treated kindly while in hospital, others were not so fortunate. For these individuals, their stay in the hospital was memorable precisely because it was such a difficult time for them. In the face of treatment from adult professionals that ranged from benevolent, sensitive, and helpful, to neglectful and callous, children nevertheless marshalled a broad range of responses and reactions.

The professional priority placed on compliance from child patients was driven by the desire to ensure their recovery from sickness and injury. Limitations on visits, attempts to include play therapy into routines, and a general tendency to prioritize efficient treatment over the comfort and sometimes compliance of the child patient, was in keeping with this. Adults who spent time in hospitals in their childhood over the early decades of the twentieth century remind us that they experienced and made sense of these adult agendas in conjunction with their own concerns, fears, and desires. While adult priorities may have been the main drivers of hospital experience, sometimes accepted (both wholeheartedly or only begrudgingly) and sometimes vociferously rejected, they never proceeded seamlessly without reaction from young patients.

6

Reforming the Body: Doctors, Educators, and Attitudes Towards Disability in Childhood

Over the early decades of the twentieth century, childhood was redefined in much professional discourse as a distinct developmental stage of life characterized, at least in part, by the need for intervention and protection. The preceding chapters explore some of the ways that medical and educational professionals contributed to these shifting emphases through their treatment of small bodies and their discursive construction of the "healthy child" over the first four decades of the twentieth century. Equally important, I have argued, are the varied responses of children and their families to medical and educational interventions. These responses add contingency and complexity to professional representations of children as vulnerable, incompetent, and unpredictable. From the perspective of the young, health and well-being flowed from lived experiences that unfolded in and took meaning primarily from the context of family, community, and culture.

Swedish reformer Ellen Key's call for the twentieth century to be (as the title of her influential book proclaimed in 1900) "the century of the child," was heartily endorsed by reformers around the world, including those in North America.[1] The "century of the child" and the new beginnings it presaged, however, traded on the end of other, less desirable childhoods. Children who ran afoul of the law, whose parents were addicted, absent, criminalized, or impoverished, who were fatherless, or racialized as non-white, became particular targets of intervention and remediation.[2] The same could be claimed for children with disabilities. From the perspective of medical and educational professionals, "the disabled child" represented uniquely difficult challenges to "good health," "normalcy," and to efforts dependent on the reformation of attitudes, behaviours, and bodies. That professionals characterized "normal" children as temporarily pathological, eventually leaving their vulnerability, incompetence, and volatility behind as they successfully matured into adults, enabled them to construct children who did not embark on this journey in conventional ways as "abnormal" or disabled. Disability, particularly intellectual but also physical, did not readily or easily yield to change.[3] For children who lived with the disability label, "the century of the child" was therefore far more ambivalent than anticipatory.

Building on my exploration thus far regarding the construction of small and young bodies, I explore here how medical and educational professionals represented disability and, more specifically, the life prospects for the disabled child through their professional writing.[4] Although they are beyond the scope of this chapter, organizations such as the Ontario Society for Crippled Children (1937–80) and Canadian branches of Easter Seals (founded in the United States in 1919) also made substantial contributions to public attitudes towards disabled children, particularly around their fundraising efforts. In the early 1920s, the Ontario Easter Seals (the first branch in Canada), brought services clubs, particularly Rotary Clubs, together to provide public information and funding for the support of children with both physical and intellectual differences. Relying on public donations, the organization held large public fundraising events for a range of projects aimed at eradicating disease or otherwise supporting treatment needs. Their first public information campaign launched in 1931 aimed to promote the universal pasteurization of milk in order to help stop the spread of tuberculosis. In 1937, Easter Seals opened the first camp for children with physical disabilities, Camp Woodeden in Komoka, Ontario. Half of the children who attended the first session of Camp Woodeden had polio. Over the century, provincial and territorial chapters of Easter Seals developed to raise funds for and awareness of the needs of children with disabilities.[5]

In the 1970s, Easter Seals, along with four other major charitable organizations in the United States began holding telethons to raise money, although Easter Seals would discontinue their use by the 1990s as criticism from the growing disability rights movement mounted. Disability scholars and activists such as Paul Longmore and Rosemarie Garland have argued that the "ritualized display of disabled people eventually develops into a cultural tradition that reinforces the ideology and power dynamics [that mark unequal relations of power between those marked as disabled and those marked as non-disabled]."[6] Other scholars have warned that cultural constructions of disability and the disabled as "in need" risk contributing to a "discourse of pity."[7] It is clear that such service organizations played significant roles in the history of children labelled with disabilities in Canada, particularly in shaping public attitudes towards them, and deserve much more critical attention from scholars. In this chapter, however, I concentrate on those doctors, nurses, and teachers who played central roles in the detection, containment, and where possible, reformation, of children with disabilities earlier in the twentieth century.[8] Solidifying a powerful partnership, medical and educational professionals utilized "dividing practices," in Michel Foucault's phrase, to identify, categorize, and improve bodies and minds judged outside the tight boundaries of "normal."[9]

Unlike their non-disabled peers, children with disabilities were not expected to leave the pathologies associated with childhood – vulnerability, incompetence, unpredictability – behind them as they grew up. Distinguished from physical disability, intellectual disability represented the most serious threat to healthy maturity. The prospects for children with intellectual disabilities were believed to be bleaker than those with physical disabilities. While medical and educational professionals, despite good intentions, constructed all disability as a threat to a healthy and normal childhood, intellectual or developmental "defectives" met primarily with resignation, pity, and fear. Judged least able to approximate "normal" behaviour, bodies, or intelligence, children with intellectual or developmental disabilities were "viewed by many health professionals as burdens both to their families and to the societies in which they lived."[10] As Nic Clarke's groundbreaking study of the treatment of "mentally deficient" children in turn-of-the century British Columbia demonstrates, however, families routinely advocated for their children, often opposing their institutionalization. They faced an uphill battle. Medical discourse, and indeed broader social attitudes, cast the mentally deficient child as incapable of growing up and therefore forever dependent on the family and the state.[11] Professionals tended to advocate detection and segregation of children judged abnormal and saw little value in providing opportunities offered to their non-disabled counterparts or even to those with physical disabilities.

The oral histories that inform this chapter are limited to those highlighting the experience of physical disability in childhood. Despite this significant limitation, these memories illuminate to some degree how professional judgments regarding "normalcy" were experienced through the body. They also underscore the family's provision of other meanings regarding physical difference beyond a focus on pathology. As the experience of Florence and Theresa (detailed in chapter 2) demonstrates, some adults who lived with polio as they grew up experienced first-hand the medical and social imperative placed on "fixing" differences through various treatment interventions. Their memories suggest that in terms of their embodied difference and their capabilities, social attitudes (centrally shaped by medical discourse) and familial attitudes could be informed by different priorities. On one hand, physical disabilities could be experienced as constraining, painful, and shameful pathologies. On the other hand, and primarily in the context of the family and communities, physical disabilities were experienced as simply another dimension of growing up. The space between these two constellations of attitudes and expectations had to be deftly mediated and navigated.[12]

While shifts in attitudes towards disability took place over the decades, underpinned by sympathetic intentions of improving and sustaining lives, I argue in this chapter that doctors, nurses, teachers, and curriculum specialists contributed in important and decisive ways to a eugenic-infused pedagogy of failure regarding disability into the 1940s and indeed beyond.[13] By casting disability as a pathological failure of the body and of the "normal" trajectory of growing up, medical and educational professionals made enduring equations between disability, abnormality, and a failed body. To different degrees and with differing options for remediation, physical and intellectual disability were thought to threaten not only the health and happiness of individual children and their families, but also public health and a stable citizenry.

EUGENICS, CONTAINMENT, AND PREVENTION IN THE CENTURY OF THE CHILD

Running through the numerous reform efforts intended to improve society and protect children at the turn of the century in Canada was an undercurrent of anxiety about threats to social order and stability. Mental and physical "deficiency" mobilized medical and educational experts in multiple national contexts at the dawn of the new century.[14] Uncertainty about the stability of the present and the future crystallized in the figure of the unproductive, morally suspect, dependent, physical, or mental "defective." Children thus labelled were not exempt from such representations, anxieties, and prejudices.

It was the so labelled "mental defective," however, who accounted for the lion's share of professional handwringing. In the early decades of the new century, professionals delivered the eugenicist message that "inferior heredity" was the principle cause of "degeneracy." Poor environments exacerbated what inheritance had begun. Children declared "abnormal" and left unmanaged, experts argued, would see little improvement or worse. Concerned medical and educational professionals thereby called for increased surveillance and segregation.[15] Segregated and supervised training, they argued, would contain and manage the failures associated with disabilities.

Several key messages about the poor life prospects of "defective" children and the threat they posed to the wider community and nation found repeated expression in the professional writing of medical and educational experts. Motivated by their belief in eugenics, leading medical figures such as Charles Kirk Clarke, dean of the Faculty of Medicine at the University of Toronto and co-founder of the Canadian National Committee for Mental Hygiene; Helen MacMurchy, Ontario's leading public health expert and inspector of the feeble-minded; and David Brankin, superintendent of British Columbia's provincial Department of Neglected Children discussed the causes of abnormality and advocated identifying, classifying, and ultimately segregating children with disabilities. A public lecture delivered to teacher candidates in 1899 by Charles Kirk Clarke exemplified these goals and attitudes. Entitled "The Evolution of Imbecility," Clarke's lecture served two purposes. First, it offered a detailed accounting of then-current medical understanding of the etiology and characteristics of "mental abnormality." Second, and importantly, Clarke encouraged teachers to do more to help "defectives" by identifying deficiencies and differentiating among their students.[16] "The more one studies heredity," Clarke asserted, "the more one is satisfied that the progressive teacher will adopt a system of teaching founded on the capabilities of the individual pupils, rather than on the theory that all children are alike and able to develop in the same direction."[17] For proponents of the institutionalization of "defectives," such as MacMurchy, Clarke, and Gordon S. Mundie, a psychiatric specialist at the Royal Victoria Hospital in Montreal, etiological discussions supported arguments for segregation and institutionalization. In his essay, "The Mentally Defective," published in the *Canadian Medical Association Journal* in 1914, Dr Mundie, made his disposition very clear:

> In Canada very little has been done for the mental defective, and in our own province of Quebec, it does not need the trained eye of the expert to see that there are large numbers of these poor unfortunates who are a menace to the stability of the country, and I have no hesitation in saying that it would be cheaper for the province to have institutions to look after them than to have them roam at large as at present.[18]

For Mundie, like other eugenic-minded health reformers, few options were reasonably available to "poor unfortunates," given conventional wisdom about the causes of mental deficiency. While sympathetic to their plight, Mundie was also clear that they were potentially dangerous and disruptive to society and needed to be contained. David Brankin, superintendent of the provincial Department of Neglected Children told his audience of women from the Girl's Central School in Victoria, British Columbia in 1920, "the problem of defective children is due to several main causes, not the least amongst these is the unjust legacy handed down by unwise parents."[19] Thus, deficiencies were believed to be the result of either a primary cause, inferior heredity being the most important example, or a secondary cause from unfavourable environmental conditions, such as birth injury, tuberculosis, fever, or syphilis. In each instance, but especially in the case of inferior heredity, little change in an otherwise bleak outlook for the afflicted was to be reasonably expected. Institutionalization afforded protection that ran both ways – for the "defective" child and, as importantly, for the public at large. Given such negative assumptions embedded in eugenic discourse, anxieties about the declining birth rate of upper- and middle-class families and the increasing birth rate of the "lower orders," including non-white immigrants, were sufficient to spark fears of race suicide amongst elites.[20]

By the 1930s, supporters of eugenics, increasingly weary of unchecked immigration in the era of the Great Depression, aggressively defended sterilization of "defectives" as the most logical preventative measure. Although the eugenics movement reached its zenith in the United States and the rest of Canada in the 1930s, hospitals for the "feeble-minded" in the western province of Alberta continued their program of forced sterilizations into the 1950s and 1960s.[21] Eugenic sterilization in most parts of Canada, however, was falling rapidly out of favour as medical professionals questioned its effectiveness and, as the atrocities of the Holocaust emerged, distanced themselves from its horrific implications.[22]

The identification, classification, and segregation of "defective" children advocated by medical and educational professionals did not go uncontested. Nic Clarke, Jessa Chupik, and David Wright have shown that many families did not want to lose their children, regardless of their disability. The institutionalization of their sons and daughters was often the last resort after all other avenues of care and family support were thoroughly exhausted. From the perspective of some parents whose children were recommended to the Orillia Asylum in Ontario, for example, "idiocy" was a curable and treatable condition requiring energy and patience. Families refused to see their children as hopeless and instead availed themselves of a range of treatment and supervisory options. Orphanages, philanthropic organizations, industrial schools, and Children's Aid Societies took in children on both a limited and on-going basis in order to relieve exhausted and financially strapped parents.[23]

The detection and containment of children with disabilities was supplemented by an increasingly robust preventative orientation in the interwar period as more finely calibrated Foucauldian "dividing practices" gained legitimacy. This was applied most particularly in the case of physical disabilities or differences. Doctors, in particular, began the search for any abnormalities long before the child was school age. Pediatric practitioners were encouraged to diagnose "degeneracy" in infants and to put the spotlight on faulty parenting (particularly on the part of mothers) as a possible causal or exasperating factor. Infants, suggested Hector Charles Cameron, bore the stamp of "inherited neuropathy" in unpleasant physical characteristics that the doctor was instructed to pathologize: "thin, meager, and tense, with rigid face and limbs ... the response to the approach of a friendly face is not a smile, but a cry or frown."[24] Lloyd P. MacHaffie, school medical officer for Ottawa's public schools, chastised parents and fellow doctors alike for the neglect of "preventative pediatrics." In 1937, MacHaffie wrote, "I am convinced, as the result of several years' examinations of thousands of school children, that a great many children enter school saddled with defects which should never have developed if adequate attention and supervision had been given during the preschool period."[25]

The number and orientation of nationwide child health centres testified to the shift towards preventative health treatment for the young. Ontario's minister of health, Dr Charles Hastings, opened the first child health centre in 1915 in Toronto to provide mothers without a family physician the "benefits of regular medical supervision."[26] By 1940, the city boasted twenty-three centres while "practically every city and town throughout the dominion had set up similar agencies for the care of the Canadian child."[27] Far beyond simply providing accessible health care, however, the centres joined public schools as important surveillance sites: "Defects are caught in over forty-five percent of the children between the ages of two and five attending the centers [sic], which otherwise, unless corrected, might handicap them for life."[28] That many "handicaps" could be caught and corrected put the onus squarely on those in positions of authority to act decisively. "Now," Dr Harris McPhedran declared in the CMAJ in 1929, "a new era is dawning and the physician of the future will be regarded chiefly as one called upon to prevent disability and disease."[29] Rather than concentrating merely on identifying "defective" children, medical and educational professionals concentrated instead on preventing and eliminating "defects."

When the opportunity to "fix" children with disabilities was either missed or not forthcoming at the level of child health centres or schools, surgery was the solution. At Toronto's HSC, the surgical repair of cleft lips and palates were common procedures that took stamina, particularly on the part of young patients. In 1934, for example, a thirteen-year-old Kitchener, Ontario girl was admitted for her eighth time. She was first admitted at two months for surgery, and for the next six years, endured yearly operations to repair her lip and palate. The previous seven surgeries, her patient record noted, "had not been completely satisfactory and she is returning for further plastic surgery."[30] Katherine Bonner, born in Terrace, British Columbia in 1945, remembered undergoing operations to correct her flat feet. She wore plaster casts on her legs for six months and endured painful infections as a result. In her experience, surgery significantly worsened her physical mobility:

> People could see me from a mile away. As soon as they saw me they knew who I was because of the way I walked right after that operation because things weren't right ... my parents really felt that doctors were gods then. You know that's where they put them – up on a pedestal.[31]

The status and power of medical science, the high social cost attached to embodied difference, and the deference given to medical doctors, as her experience made clear, tended to encourage compliance.

SCHOOLING FOR DISABILITY?

By the beginning of the First World War, schooling in the form of manual training was held out as an important bulwark against the threats associated with unmanaged "abnormal" youngsters. The arrival of large numbers of non-white immigrants, particularly at end of the First World War, was seen as a threat to the country's dominant British identity. Public schools, as they had done in the case of physical and mental "abnormality," were called upon to inculcate "healthy citizenship" by promoting assimilation. Alberta school medical inspector, Dr J. Dunn, echoed widespread sentiment in this regard:

> We are educating a nation. It rests with us to say whether ... the race shall advance or retreat. [In the] public schools ... the children come together and mingle ... here they begin to understand the nature of British citizenship. If, therefore, we wish to produce and perpetuate a nation of strong, virile, intellectual, and normal men and women, let us see to it that our public schools are in every way of the best possible character.[32]

Physical and mental "defectives," or "cripples," as they were described in professional discourse, were at the very centre of debates and contestations regarding public health and school reform as they evolved over the early to mid-decades of the century. As Jason Ellis, Angus McLaren, Gerald Thompson, and Nic Clarke have shown, Canadian medical and educational professionals influenced by eugenic theories on race betterment routinely looked to schools and other major social institutions as partners against unidentified and, more importantly, untreated and untrained "feeble-minded" and physically "defective" youngsters.[33] Perfectly positioned to disseminate new curricular information about physical and mental hygiene, schools emerged as comprehensive human sorting stations: large numbers of children, compelled to attend, could be tested, examined, and sorted into "normal" or "abnormal" categories, and treatment, if indicated, pursued.

Concern for the proper surveillance of "defective" children was shared by those more directly involved in the public schools, such as school medical inspectors, curricula developers for teachers and students, and teachers themselves. Influential leaders such as Vancouver's supervisor of subnormal classes, Josephine Dauphinee,[34] were preoccupied with imparting lessons in health and hygiene, particularly targeting abstinence from alcohol and tobacco, as critical ways to address suspected causes of "abnormality."

Ideas about heredity in school textbooks, first introduced in chapter 4, bear repeating here. Dr A.P. Knight, professor of physiology at Queen's University in Kingston, Ontario and author of *The Ontario Public School Hygiene*, wrote,

> If you have followed the teachings of this book thus far, it must be clear to you now that our lives from birth until old age are shaped largely by two great influences: (1) by what we inherit from our parents, grandparents, or other ancestral relatives, and (2) by our environment, that is, by our surroundings."[35]

Gordon S. Mundie argued that while parental inheritance was no doubt important, inferior environments could have equally tragic and regrettable effects on children's health. Much was at stake for advocates of improved standards of public health and hygiene. "A condition of ill health, actual disease, or starvation of the mother," Mundie reminded his readers, "cannot but be injurious to the growing embroyo [sic], and the same may be said of improper food, impure air, deficient light, and inadequate sleep, which are so often the lot of young children in our city slums."[36] Regardless of causation, outcomes were similar: "mental deficiency is a defect of the higher centres, not a disease," Mundie made clear. "Therefore, there is no cure for it."[37]

In his 1916 address to the Alberta Medical Association, Dr D.J. Dunn spoke from his additional experience as medical inspector of schools in Edmonton. In Dunn's experience, physical "defects" were just as troublesome, both for individual children and society as a whole, as mental "defects." Bad teeth, for example, set in motion a costly chain of debilitating, but ultimately preventable, events. He warned that

> decayed teeth mean aching teeth, aching teeth mean germ-ridden mouths and germ-saturated food favouring the propagation of contagious diseases, poor mastication and digestion, impaired nourishment and bodily resistance, intestinal and general toxic

absorption, all of which prevent proper intellectual advancement, and favour the various forms of physical disturbances and degeneration."[38]

For Dunn, like other professionals, the primary benefit of compulsory public schooling was as a sorting station for "normal" and "abnormal" children. "Normal" youngsters progressed through their grades, "abnormal" youngsters were, depending on their distance from "normalcy," either treated and improved or segregated into special classes or institutions. The segregation of "subnormal" children in special classes had begun in earnest first in France with the work of Edward Sequin, onward to Germany, and by the turn of the twentieth century had become established practice in Cleveland, Chicago, and New York.[39] By 1910, authorities in Toronto were identifying and segregating "subnormal" children. Two pieces of Canadian legislation further facilitated the impulse to identify, classify, and segregate the "abnormal": the *Special Class Act* of 1911 and the *Auxiliary Class Act* of 1914.[40] Helen MacMurchy, a leading proponent of the legislation, praised the main provisions of the act which allowed not only for special classes in the public school buildings, but also empowered school boards to build separate institutions, such as Industrial Training Schools and Farm Colonies for the Mentally Defective. The latter were particularly important in MacMurchy's estimation for they "provide protection for the mentally defective and renders them as happy and as useful as they can be; it also protects the community and the nation."[41]

School and public health work satisfied two interrelated impulses: to protect and enhance the welfare of children labelled "deficient" and to protect society from the dangers such children were assumed to represent. Laying the foundations of an enduring pedagogy of failure, experts in this period characterized physical and mental disability as the irrevocable corruption of body and moral fibre. In 1915, Dr Mundie underlined this enduring link between "defects" and costs to the community:

> Crime, like all conduct, is an attribute of mental life and this being so, in order to get at the cause of crime we must study the

mental life of the criminal. Very little has been done in developing this science, but what has been done has clearly shown that most criminals are physically and mentally inferior.[42]

Children thus afflicted and not properly dealt with, warned Helen MacMurchy, "cannot make good in the community ... and are a source of evil and a burden of expense."[43]

While leading medical professionals like Mundie and MacMurchy characterized segregation of "defectives" as beneficial to the interests of the nation, teachers working in public schools acknowledged more personal benefits. One Ontario teacher, writing to fellow intermediate grade teachers in 1915, pointed out that the *Auxiliary Class Act* made possible the temporary segregation of a whole range of students thought both ill-served in classrooms for "normal" youngsters and destined to hold back the progress of peers:

> These [auxiliary classes] may be established under the Act for foreigners: handicapped by language, manners, habits – better be taught by an expert who could more rapidly pass them on as they are often possessed of mature ability; Japanese, Chinese, Russian, Italian, semi-deaf, semi-blind, physically defective, crippled, some so much so that they have to be carried or have to climb long flights of stairs on their knees.[44]

The conflation between racialized "handicap" ("foreigners" believed to be handicapped by language, manners, habits) with physical "handicap" suggests the extent to which "normalcy" was socially constructed by those in positions powerful enough to influence attitudes, beliefs, and policy.[45]

While attendance at public school became compulsory over the early decades of the twentieth century, some children with disabilities found it difficult to attend school on a regular basis. Surgery, compromised mobility, or bullying could make attendance difficult or dreaded. In the case of Florence Drake,[46] born in Vancouver in 1908 and struck with polio at the age of two, hospitalization severely compromised school attendance. Between the ages of eleven and fourteen, she spent most of her time in hospital undergoing painful treatments and a series of operations in hopes of "normalizing" her condition. Her lack of conventional mobility rendered her unable to attend school for years at a time.[47] Theresa Elliott[48] recalled that a helpful neighbour and a sympathetic principal were key to her success at school. Born in 1920 in Parry Sound, Ontario, she did not attend school until she was ten years old, and only then with considerable effort:

> I remember living in the country and in winter it was very slippery – I couldn't get to school – I couldn't balance myself. And there was a boy next door who was from a big family. And do you know that every morning when it was slippery he would bring his sleigh and try to get me to school ... I was never counted late by the principal if I got there and it was slippery. Because he knew I couldn't manage like the rest of them, and I couldn't keep my balance like the rest of them.[49]

In an era before accommodation imperatives, children with disabilities relied on a network of allies – including families, neighbours, and school officials – to help them get to, and remain at, school. If goodwill was not forthcoming or available, regular attendance at school could prove elusive.

Peers, inside and outside school, acted as powerful agents of exclusion for some children with disabilities. Within the culture of childhood, the pedagogy of failure was also policed and enforced. Agnes Lockhart, born in 1939 and raised in Neepawa, Manitoba, found school attendance difficult because she was made to feel like an outsider there. She dreaded school but found some refuge in summer camp attendance: "But I did get sent to crippled children's camp one time, and this was wonderful. I had never been to camp ... I wasn't a freak there, you know, because everybody there was odd. I even got to have an upper bunk."[50] As a student at North Vancouver High School in British Columbia in the late 1930s, Robin Williams remembered "brains and a winning personality were valued, but among boys prowess at sports was probably number one."[51] Athletic competition was seen as the quintessential way to display those attributes perceived to be the rightful domain of young and virile male bodies – strength, speed, agility and muscularity.[52] Williams was acutely aware of the importance of sports since he was for the most part excluded from them. Having survived poliomyelitis, he spent much of his childhood judged unable to compete with his brothers and friends. They, unlike him, easily satisfied gendered expectations about the physical abilities of "normal" boys.

Girls were not exempt from such gendered discussions. Conventional understandings of "beauty" precluded bodies that were considered in any way "abnormal." In a 1939 health textbook approved for use in Canadian schools, health was similarly linked with "good looks" via strong, tall bodies in the case of girls. "Mary is a healthy girl," students were taught, because "she stands straight and tall ... she gains in weight and grows taller ... Mary is a pretty girl because she is such a healthy girl."[53] Theresa Elliott, profiled in chapter 2 and who developed a "limp" as a result of her poliomyelitis, learned as she grew up that she would simply never be considered an attractive mate. Certainly the actions of her father, in conjunction with a larger culture of prejudice, reinforced her feelings as an undesirable, even imperilled, outsider: "My dad always had the idea that because I was lame, that someone would take advantage of me. And he was very strict. I remember right up until I was sixteen, I could only go out on Friday night and I had to be in by nine, and if I wasn't in by nine my dad was out looking for me."[54] While girls in general were often held to close account by adults, based on their liability for domestic labour as well as assumptions about their sexual vulnerability, those labelled with a disability were doubly burdened.

Approved health curriculum on the eve of the Second World War made schools both implicit and explicit contributors to the failure associated with physical and mental "defects." While the explicit emphasis on eugenics and heredity no longer took centre stage, potent links between "normal" bodies and civic pride and purpose were forged. Good health, signalled most immediately by "normal" vigorous young bodies, demonstrated democratic citizenship. A "failed" body continued to signal a "failed" nation. Although progressive health curriculum prided itself on being innovative and cutting edge ("the aim of the new schools is learning to live"), long-standing elements of a pedagogy of failure endured. Self-control continued to influence how children and young adults were encouraged to think about their embodied selves. "No matter what you wish to do in the world," suggested J. Mace Andress and Elizabeth Breeze in *Health Essentials in High School* (1938), "your ability to control your own mind and muscles must be the basis of your success."[55] Health, according to Andress and Breeze, was a commodity easily won if students were willing to "first, have a desire to be healthy; secondly have the determination to undergo training in order to win health." Students were taught that "most people could win health if they only knew how and tried."[56] In a 1939 textbook vignette involving an exchange between a student named Martha and her teacher, Miss Long, internalized discipline of a compliant body was implicitly connected to success in life: "I heard the bell in the hall and I just jumped," said Martha. "I wanted to run. But the rule for a fire drill is 'walk, don't run.' So I told my muscles to make me walk." "Your muscles wanted to run," said Miss Long, "but you told them not to run. Good muscles will do what you tell them to do."[57]

As Miss Long's approval of Martha's embodied restraint insinuates, disciplined, compliant bodies housed good children. Students able to master and control their bodies to benefit from "good muscles" were on the road to successful adulthood, the ultimate goal of childhood in the eyes of many adults. The implications of this kind of discourse for children with bodies or behaviours that marked them as "abnormal" was, however, very problematic.

With the onset of the Second World War, psychology became an increasingly influential force in the medical treatment of children labelled with physical and mental differences. Particularly as a result of military-oriented research on the suitability of recruits, battle fatigue, and the "problem" of the returning soldier, psychological reasoning increasingly shaped professional attitudes and treatment.[58] The increasing popularity of psychology as medical tool over the war years signaled at least in part a growing sensitivity to the social and emotional needs of children. It would, for example, contribute to shifting hospital practice over the next decades that acknowledged the beneficial effects of daily visiting and a play program on the mental health of young children.[59]

Children with physical and/or mental differences were often assumed to suffer negative psychological ramifications. Rather than attributing this vulnerability to larger social prejudices, medical practitioners focused on the individual and their differences as the cause. Dr Hamilton Baxter, a plastic surgeon at the Children's Memorial Hospital in Montreal, argued in 1941 that "the most important effect of protruding ears on a child is psychological and may be expressed either in a feeling of inferiority which may cause the child to avoid personal contacts, or perhaps to develop a super-abundance of self-expression in an effort to compensate an injured ego."[60] In either case, Baxter suggested to his colleagues early detection of the "defect" on the part of parents enabled corrective surgery to be carried out before any psychological damage occurred. "Children have a keen ability to detect the unusual," Baxter pointed out, "and any abnormality in a playmate is the object of frank curiosity and ridicule."[61] The presentation of physical and mental differences as the cause of ill health or social ridicule made adult professionals, unwittingly or otherwise, accomplices to the pedagogy of failure.

CONCLUSIONS

Medical and educational professionals in Canada over the first four decades of the twentieth century equated disability with a compromised, if not failed, childhood. Their characterization of "abnormal" children complimented and was predicated upon their understanding of the "normal" pathologies associated with being young and small. While "normal" children would grow up and leave these pathologies behind, "abnormal" children would not. To construct "the normal child," in other words, was to construct its "other." Their efforts to root out disability were forged on children's bodies and included various interventions to change, improve, "normalize," or simply contain intellectual and physical differences. Between 1900 and the beginning of the Second World War, doctors and educational specialists in Canada had much to say about "defective" children. While considerable shifts took place, powerful ideas about the constitution of "normal" bodies and behaviours saturated the professional discourse, drove attitudes, and shaped practices. Disability was presented through a pedagogy of failure that operated within much of the professional discourse over the period under study and indeed well beyond. While wartime doctors and educationalists no longer emphasized "inferior heredity" they continued to cast "difference" in terms of tragedy and mistake. Dr Ross Campbell, waxing poetic about the "spastic child" (i.e. child with cerebral palsy), wrote in 1946 that "it is not too unbelievable that Nature, which puts together the most intricate jigsaw puzzle imaginable, the human body, should slip up occasionally and leave a piece out."[62] Similar characterizations of the "failed child" echoed a decade later. In 1957, prominent Vancouver pediatrician and advocate for the expansion of outpatient services for children, Dr Donald Paterson, pointed out the benefits of early detection of "defects":

> It must therefore be our aim to detect the handicap as early as possible, to keep him in good health and to start rehabilitation and planning for his future at once. If this is done, it is quite surprising how many children formerly considered to have no salvage value can be made into useful citizens, wholly or partially self-supporting.[63]

The oral histories of adults who grew up with a physical difference over the period give us another perspective on professional efforts to end what was understood as unfortunate and unhealthy circumstances. While medical and educational professionals were undoubtedly motivated by a strong desire to improve the lives of children, the consequences of their efforts could effectively solidify oppressive associations between disability and "abnormality." In some cases, institutionalization or surgical solutions had the opposite effect: they compounded disabilities rather than "fixing" them. As Bill Lossky, who grew up in the early 1950s in East York, near Toronto, Ontario remembered:

> I had a cousin who, um, who they called retarded, but was probably autistic. Marilyn was pretty clever. She could do amazing stuff but she spent almost her entire life institutionalized. Marilyn was twenty-some-odd years old and they said she had the mind of a five-year-old, but she could type a hundred and forty words a minute and play the piano.[64]

Children with disabilities and their families actively navigated these often choppy waters, and despite desires to conform to social expectations and lead healthy lives, did not always heed professional advice deemed too invasive, impractical, or unhelpful. Despite the tenacity of the pedagogy of failure, many children labelled disabled carved out meaningful lives.

CONCLUSION

Small Matters: Historical Meaning and Children's Embodiment

On 23 August 1937 thirteen-year-old Harvey Bredeau came to Toronto's Hospital for Sick Children, accompanied by his father and the Indian agent. He lived with his parents on the Wikwemikong Reserve on Manitoulin Island, Ontario, one of four children, with two older brothers and a younger sister. His patient record notes that the attending doctor received a "rather inadequate" history of Harvey's health from the Indian agent but does not indicate whether Harvey or his father were also consulted.

Harvey appeared to the attending doctor to be, according to comments on his record, "a large boy with a completely destroyed nose – not acutely ill." While a handwritten version of the record stated that "his skin is excessively dirty," the typed version, presumably produced after Harvey was admitted, recorded instead that his "skin is pigmented due to Indian parentage."[1]

The record tells us that Harvey appeared to be healthy until his tenth year when an ulceration appeared in his nose. It gradually spread and deepened to involve the entire structure of the nose and "practically all the nasal septum." Not only was his overall health affected, the record noted that it caused "horrible disfigurement." Harvey was brought to the HSC to treat the underlying disease and to have plastic surgery to improve his appearance. He was immediately diagnosed with congenital syphilis and a range of secondary conditions. It was also discovered at this time that he suffered from a serious heart condition.

Without elaboration, his chart notes that he was "taken to Thistletown" on 27 August 1937. Located in Rexdale, a community northwest of Toronto, Thistletown was then a branch of the HSC that specialized in long-term care for child patients with chronic conditions, and those needing to build their health in the face of multiple surgeries. By 1957, it became Thistletown Regional Centre, the first institution devoted to children and youth with mental illness.[2] With no additional detail, Harvey's record notes that "social services is trying [underlined in original] to make arrangements for a foster home." This suggests that relations with Harvey's family had in some form broken down, or that his parents were judged unable to sufficiently care for the boy. Given the emphasis in the record on attempts to locate a home for him, success in this regard had clearly proven difficult. As Veronica Strong-Boag's work on history of fostering and adoption in Canada has shown, First Nation children, and those with physical or mental disabilities, were often the last to find families willing to welcome them. More often, they languished in the care of institutions.[3]

Between mid-March and early August of 1938, Harvey underwent nine surgeries to repair his nose and improve his breathing. No details regarding the success or failure of these multiple surgeries, nor about how Harvey fared over their course are offered in his record. On 30 August 1938 in this fourteenth year, the record states that Harvey Bredeau died from heart failure.

The details contained in Harvey Bredeau's HSC patient record, like that of Michael Londell (introduced in chapter 5), afford a particular window onto his experiences with conventional medicine, medical practitioners, and notions of good health in early twentieth-century Canada. Like the professional medical literature and textbooks explored in previous chapters, they represent a valuable source of information on attitudes of medical professionals towards their patients. From the perspective and judgment of medical staff, we learn something of Harvey's journey of diagnosis and treatment. As Wendy Mitchinson has shown in the context of women's medical treatment in nineteenth- and twentieth-century Canada, however, patient records provide some answers to particular questions but remain stubbornly silent on others.[4]

The power imbalance between Harvey and his family on one hand, and state and medical authorities on the other, for example, speaks most readily through the patient record. The observation and evaluation of Harvey's medical condition is told entirely from the perspective of medical staff. That the Indian agent was called upon to supply Harvey's history, that medical staff judged him to be a large boy, not acutely ill, but suffering from a "horrible disfigurement," is relayed without indication that Harvey or his family were consulted. From the point of view of those in charge, his condition demanded multiple diagnoses, interventions, and an extended stay under medical supervision. The paternalistic role performed by the Indian agent and the observation by medical staff that his skin was "excessively dirty," replaced with "skin is pigmented due to Indian heritage" in a typed version of the record, suggests that race mattered in Harvey's interactions with staff, although to what degree is not clearly articulated in the record. Finally, although the record holds no details about the reasons for Harvey's referral to social services for foster care, the surveillance of children and families deemed at odds with white, middle-class values was commonplace. This was especially true in the case of First Nation families, into which the patriarchal state in general, and particularly Western medicine, have a long history of intervention, both benevolent and malevolent.[5]

Like others with histories of subordination and exclusion from social power, such as women, Indigenous peoples, the working class, people with disabilities, people from non-white racial backgrounds, and children and young people, share in the experience of being told what to be, what to do, how to act, what to think, and where to go, by more powerful others. By virtue first and foremost of their young age and small size relative to adults, children have been largely conceptualized as temporary entities on their way to becoming something more desirable: productive, virtuous, and well-adjusted women and men. The teleological notion of the child as a projection into the future, as Claudia Castaneda argues, a "conceptualization of the child as a potentiality rather than an actuality," has been a considerable force shaping the historical experience of children and youth.[6]

To answer our questions about the experience of children such as Harvey Bredeau and Michael Londell we must ask questions that complicate and shift the traditional focus on the power imbalance between youngsters and adults, lay persons and professionals. The oral histories highlighted in this book afford new ways to understand the power differentials between generations, how they were choreographed and structured in the past. They also shed considerable light on how young people maintained, challenged, and transformed relationships.

The childhood memories of Florence, Marc, Alice, and Theresa explored in chapter 2, and Shirley, Lily, Jack, and Lily explored in chapter 3, for example, indicate that medicine and health were thoroughly mediated discourses in family life. Far from simply "imposed from above," the dictates of doctors, nurses, and teachers were, as I demonstrate in chapters highlighting the experience of children in hospital and school, variously accepted, rejected, ignored, exalted, misunderstood, welcomed, and despised. Encounters with professional medical practitioners (rare or even non-existent in the experience of some youngsters) were positive and negative, or some combination of both, resulting in improved health for some children and compromised health and social disadvantage for others. Children and their families, in other words, braided their various encounters with medicine, medical treatment, and formal and informal education about health and their bodies into other strands of experience that constituted their childhoods.

The oral history of Amelia Desjardin once again illustrates the complex meanings, apart from formal encounters with doctors and nurses, which health, sickness, and the body held for the young. Amelia was born in 1920 in Monteau, a small village in northern Quebec.[7] She lost her father when she was three years old to a heart attack and was raised primarily by her mother. Her mother did eventually remarry, but her stepfather worked away from home for months at a time clearing bush for roads. While her stepfather was well paid for his work, a great deal of the family budget, Amelia recalled, was put towards his alcohol consumption. The family eventually expanded to include Amelia and four half-siblings: two sisters and two brothers.

When Amelia was fourteen years old, one of her brothers, then five years, complained of a sore throat. The doctor visited the family, a source of some stress, according to Amelia, since the family budget was tight. The doctor gave the boy only a package of lozenges. She confided that the doctor's treatment went unchallenged by her family, even though they suspected that it was not adequate. Their suspicions were bore out the next day. The boy's throat was swollen "all the way from his chin to his chest," Amelia remembered. Her mother left to make the long journey with her brother to the nearest hospital, leaving Amelia in charge of her three younger siblings. Her afflicted brother died shortly after they arrived at the hospital. Amelia's mother, in a state of shock and grief, was admitted and remained hospitalized for two subsequent weeks. In the meantime, the family home was quarantined.

Catapulted to the role of parent to her younger siblings, Amelia recalled being by turns terrified to be alone without adult support, worried about the specter of diphtheria, but determined to carry out the responsibilities thrust upon her. She recalled that lighting a reluctant and finicky wood stove in the morning to provide heat and keep the water pipes from freezing became a daily priority for her. She took each day as it came, ensuring that her siblings stayed healthy, warm, and fed.

The finer details of everyday life during the ordeal, however, were not emphasized in Amelia's oral history memories. Instead, she shared her thoughts about the loss of her brother and its meaning in her family history:

> My father, when he came home, because his son was dead, you know, he drank more. So it was not very pleasant. And I was worried for my mother, too. So when she came home it was nice. She was such a good mother. I don't really have bad memories. For having so many problems, and so many hard times, I still remember most that she was so good to us. But she really had a difficult time too – about that death. He was a special little boy, too. He was so cute.[8]

Amelia's discussion of her brother's illness and death focused on the ramifications of the tragedy for her family and their ability to cope and endure. She was relieved when her mother returned home, but greatly concerned for her emotional well-being. Her stepfather's increased drinking added to the instability caused by grief and loss. Despite these challenges, however, Amelia emphasizes that her family survived, primarily due to the strength and affection of her mother. In Amelia's recollections, the challenges posed by her brother's illness and death went to the very heart of familial cohesiveness and stability. It had personal ramifications that extended to Amelia herself, as she faced the daunting task of parenting her siblings on her own in the midst of quarantine.

Childhood memories relayed through oral histories like that of Amelia's are imperfect forums for child perspectives on health and illness. They nevertheless get us closer to an approach that assumes that children made a difference in the way change unfolded in the past. Recalling their child selves, participants revealed how they felt about, coped with, ignored, and challenged the priorities of medical and educational professionals. They also suggest that, in the experience of some, sickness and health was only tangentially influenced by professional interventions and, instead, gained much more important meaning in domestic and community domains.

Medical and educational professionals, nevertheless, did produce powerful knowledge about children and their bodies. Changes in professional medical approaches to illness, from an emphasis on containing contagion, to insistence on compliance with the expertise of professionals, to a preventative approach in which professionals were conceptualized as the sole arbitrators of health, had complex consequences for the young. Small and young bodies, according to doctors and nurses, had unique pathological characteristics that distinguished them from more healthful adult norms. The assumption of children's natural physical pathologies lent support for character traits associated with the young: vulnerability, innocence, incompetence, and unpredictability. The construction of children's bodies alongside racialized, classed, gendered, and able-bodied ideas about the "healthy child" influenced how children were treated and what they learned.

Moving beyond a traditional focus on powerful adults and powerless children, this book explores how encounters with medical and educational professionals, discursive and otherwise, shaped generational relationships, what role race, gender, class, and disability played, and how young people responded to, mitigated, and transformed these relationships. Most importantly, by foregrounding childhood memories of sickness and health, I've emphasized that relationships between generations were not simply hierarchical and oppositional but were thoroughly negotiated, dynamic, and contingent. In pursuing this line of inquiry, I have taken seriously Robert MacIntosh's argument that

> the history of childhood has been constructed through studies of adults and their activities – and children's responses to these. Only rarely is the agency of children recognized in the historical literature: children tend to be portrayed as passive beings who are the objects of welfare and educational strategies. The history of childhood becomes the history of the efforts of others on children's behalf.[9]

Employing the lens of children's medical treatment and health education, and a theoretical approach that evokes size and age as important interpretative categories, I've explored how children themselves experienced sickness and health. This perspective places a spotlight on what children learned about themselves and their place in their family and broader community as they grew up.

In contemporary times, the health and well-being of children, and particularly young children, still preoccupy government, professionals, and parents. A mountain of empirical evidence gathered by governmental, non-governmental, and non-profit groups over the past twenty years suggest that while the majority of youngsters in Canada enjoy robust health, barriers based on factors such as race and class continue to disadvantage certain children.[10] Poverty is recognized as the main challenge to equitable health status amongst children in the Canadian context and has drawn both concern and criticism, and neglect and indifference from local, national, and international bodies.[11]

Despite continued inaction on the part of the federal Conservative government led by Prime Minister Stephen Harper, demands to address social inequality in Canada continue to be made. In their 2009 report, *In from the Margins: A Call to Action on Poverty, Housing and Homelessness*, the Standing Senate Committee on Social Affairs, Science, and Technology added their voice. They demanded that

> the federal government adopt as a core social policy poverty eradication and that all programmes dealing with poverty and homelessness are to lift Canadians out of poverty rather than make living within poverty more manageable and that the federal government work with the provinces and territories to adopt a similar goal.[12]

Despite such demands, levels of poverty in Canada, a rich nation, continue to be high, with the province of British Columbia outpacing the rest of the country. In his 1998 annual report on the health of British Columbians, then-provincial medical health officer, Dr John Millar, complained that "it's shocking that in a wealthy province there is not enough money for proper nutrition." Children from single parent families, First Nations, and those in northern communities, Millar reported, were twice as likely to live in poverty or to suffer early death than those living in more urbanized areas of the province.[13] In 2010, unacceptably high levels of children continue to live in poverty, with those from the most marginalized populations suffering the most.[14]

The history explored in this book provides meaningful insight into these long-standing barriers to equity. Children from non-white and/or poor families, like Marc Trapier and Shirley Brand, lacked many of the opportunities to enrich and protect their health status afforded to their white and middle-class contemporaries. Youngsters had a wide range of experiences with medical and educational professionals, some proved to be positive and life enriching while others resulted in the opposite. In all cases, they brought their own priorities and concerns to bear on these experiences. Like young people in the present, the children profiled in this book interacted with health and welfare professionals firmly within the broader context of their families and communities and in concert with the rhythms and needs of both. When a health crisis occurred, the consequences, as is the case today, reached out beyond patient, to parents, siblings, and community. For children in the past and the present, confronting death and disease, managing relationships with doctors, nurses, teachers, and parents, learning to be healthy (and staying that way), was and is no small matter.

APPENDICES

APPENDIX ONE

Causes of Infant Death in Canada, for five-year periods, 1921–50*

	Cardio-vascular renal diseases	Influenza, bronchitis, and pneumonia+	Diseases of early infancy+	Tuberculosis	Cancer	Gastritis, duodenitis, enteritis and colitis	Accidents	Communicable diseases■
1946–1950	414.0	55.3	58.3	37.1	129.3	14.2	58.9	4.9
1941–1945	403.3	69.1	57.2	50.1	123.3	19.2	60.6	9.7
1936–1940	337.6	97.5	60.2	56.2	113.8	24.1	55.9	15.6
1931–1935	297.5	100.6	74.5	65.5	100.9	35.4	52.4	17.8
1926–1930	273.1	133.8	97.7	80.3	88.0	54.9	58.8	35.0
1921–1925	221.9	141.1	111.0	85.1	75.9	72.2	51.5	47.1

(Average annual rates per 100,000 live births)

* Excerpted from Statistics Canada, Series B-35-50, "Average annual number of deaths and death rates for leading causes of death, Canada, for five-year periods, 1921 to 1974."
+ Pneumonia of newborn included in both "diseases of early infancy" and "influenza, bronchitis, and pneumonia" for all years (except for the province of Quebec, 1921 to 1925).
■ Includes diphtheria, whooping cough, measles, scarlet fever, typhoid fever.

APPENDIX TWO

Participant Information

Name (alphabetical order)	Sex	Year of birth	Place of birth	Race/ethnicity*	Child Health Project (CHP)
Katherine Bonner	Female	1945	Terrace, BC	Anglo-Saxon	017
Shirley Brand	Female	1924	Deseronto, Ontario	Chippewa/Mohawk	1
John Brennan	Male	1942	North York, Ontario	Anglo-Celtic	14
Mark Cameron	Male	1926	Penticton, BC	Anglo-Saxon	20
Mattie Clarke	Female	1913	Winnipeg, Manitoba	Anglo-Saxon	O4N
Lina Colussi	Female	1926	Kelowna, BC	Italian	32
Eileen Davies	Female	1943	Barrie, Ontario	Anglo-Saxon	03N
Janie Dearland	Female	1930	Saskatoon, Saskatchewan	Anglo-Celtic	18N
Amelia Desjardin	Female	1920	Monteau, Quebec	French-Canadian	013
Florence Drake	Female	1908	Vancouver, BC	Anglo-Saxon	023
Theresa Elliott	Female	1920	Parry Sound, Ontario	Anglo-Saxon	10
Irena Friedman	Female	1945	New Brunswick	German Jew	2
Megumi Itou	Female	1941	Ocean Falls, BC	Japanese (Okinawan)	40
Frank Johnson	Male	1953	Sugar Cane, BC	Shuswap	02N
Andrea Knott	Female	1918	Stoughton, Saskatchewan	Anglo-Saxon	11N

Appendices

Name (alphabetical order)	Sex	Year of birth	Place of birth	Race/ethnicity*	Child Health Project (CHP)
Agnes Lockhart	Female	1939	Gladstone, Manitoba	Anglo-Saxon	24
Bill Lossky	Male	1949	East York, Ontario	Anglo-Saxon	015
Doris MacKenzie	Female	1943	Montreal, Quebec	Anglo-Saxon	22
Lily Mason	Female	1925	Fort Pelly, Saskatchewan	Cree	4
Alice Mercer	Female	1916	Montreal, Quebec	Anglo-Celtic	5
Kyle Moss	Male	1946	Peterborough, Ontario	Anglo-Saxon	007N
Glenda Myers	Female	1910	Halifax, NS	Anglo-Saxon	10N
Jack McCrea	Male	1926	Huntsville, Ontario	Anglo-Saxon	7A
Trisha Price	Female	1948	Kelowna, BC	Anglo-Saxon	19
Jenny Randall	Female	1927	Penticton, BC	Anglo-Saxon	29N
Gladys Rupert	Female	1944	Port Sydney, Ontario	Anglo-Saxon	011
Kathryn Sutherland	Female	1927	Toronto, Ontario	Anglo-Saxon	06N
William Sweeney	Male	1948	Ottawa, Ontario	Anglo-Celtic	008N
Catherine Tilley	Female	1935	Bing Inlet, Ontario	Anglo-Saxon	8
Marc Trapier	Male	1913	Hochelaga-Maisonneuve, Quebec	French-Canadian	024
Donald Traster	Male	1950	Brockville, Ontario	Anglo-Celtic	6
Monica Welsh	Female	1921	Abbotsford, BC	Anglo-Celtic	021N

* Participants self-identified their racial or ethnic heritage.

APPENDIX THREE

My Health Record

Name _____ School _____
Grade _____ Teacher _____

Directions: (1) Count one for every point of the Daily Health Program you have kept each day. (2) Pupils who are up to average weight who are gaining properly may have credit for milk and rest at school, without taking them. (3) Add one point for four glasses of water drunk between meals. (4) Count one off for each of these health faults: (a) Putting pencils in the mouth or anything except for eating, drinking, or cleaning teeth. (b) Sneezing or coughing without using handkerchief. (c) Going a whole day without going to toilet. (d) Eating candy or pickles between meals. (e) Drinking stimulating drinks such as tea, coffee, and coca-cola.

Wash
Clean teeth
Milk for breakfast
Cereal for breakfast
Fruit for breakfast
Milk at school
Rest at school
Out-door play after school

Wash for supper
Milk for supper
Fruit or green vegetables
Stay at home all evening
Clean teeth
Bed at (7-8-9)
Sleep with open windows
Score for day (20 is perfect)

Weight

Source: J. Mace Andress, *Wide-Awake School* (Boston: Ginn and Company, 1931), 33.

Notes

INTRODUCTION

1 All names of oral history participants quoted in this book have been changed. Child Health Project (CHP), Interview 04N, transcript, 3.
2 CHP, Interview 8, transcript, 7–8.
3 CHP, Interview 40, transcript, 16–7.
4 CHP, Interview 14, transcript, 1–7.
5 On the construction of children's bodies in the past see Gleason, "Race, Class, and Health"; Gleason, "Disciplining the Student Body"; Gleason, "Embodied Negotiations."
6 Little, 'No car, no radio, no liquor permit'; Ursel, *Private Lives, Public Policy*; Christie, *Engendering the State: Family, Work, and Welfare in Canada*.
7 Veronica Strong-Boag, "Getting to Now: Children in Distress in Canada's Past," in Wharf, *Community Approaches to Child Welfare*, 29–46.
8 The literature in Canada, America, and Europe in this regard is vast. Some key and classic works that helped shape our understanding of children and youth during the era of twentieth-century welfare reform include: Sutherland, *Children in English-Canadian Society*; Joseph Kett, *Rites of Passage: Adolescence in America, 1790 to the Present* (New York: Basic Books, 1977); Steven L. Schlossman, *Love and the American Delinquent: The Theory and Practice of "Progressive" Juvenile Justice, 1825–1920* (Chicago: University of Chicago Press, 1977); Paula Fass, *The Damned and the Beautiful: American Youth in the 1920s* (New York: Oxford University Press, 1977); Lewis, "Creating the Little Machine"; Linda Pollock, *Forgotten Children: Parent-child Relations from 1500 to 1900* (Cambridge: Cambridge University Press, 1983); Zelizer, *Pricing the*

Priceless Child; Linda Gordon, *Heroes of Their Own Lives – A History of Family Violence, Boston, 1880–1960* (New York: Viking, 1988); Hugh Cunningham, *Children of the Poor: Representations of Childhood Since the Seventeen Century* (Cambridge: Blackwell, 1991); Comacchio, *Nations are Built of Babies*; Joy Parr, *Labouring Children: British Immigrant Apprentices to Canada, 1896–1924* (Toronto: University of Toronto Press, 1994); Harvey Graff, *Conflicting Paths: Growing Up in America* (Cambridge, MA: Harvard University Press, 1995); Neil Sutherland, *Growing Up: Childhood in English Canada from the Great War to the Age of Television* (Toronto: University of Toronto Press, 1997); Steven Mintz, *Huck's Raft: A History of American Childhood* (Cambridge, MA: Belknap Press of Harvard University Press, 2004); Dominique Marshall (translated by Nicola Doone Danby) *The Social Origins of the Welfare State: Québec Families, Compulsory Education and Family Allowances, 1940–1955* (Waterloo: Wilfrid Laurier Press, 2006).

9 Alvin Finkle, *Social Policy and Practice in Canada: A History* (Waterloo: Wilfrid Laurier Press, 2006), 169–72.

10 See Sutherland, *Children in English-Canadian Society*; Veronica Strong-Boag, *The New Day Recalled: Lives of Girls and Women in English Canada, 1919–39* (Markham: Copp Clark Pitman, 1988); Angus McLaren, *Our Own Master Race: Eugenics in Canada, 1885–1945* (Toronto: McClelland and Stewart, 1990); Mariana Valverde, *The Age of Light, Soap and Water* (Toronto: McClelland and Stewart, 1991); Stern and Markel, *Formative Years*; Comacchio, *Nations are Built of Babies*; Roger Cooter, ed., *In the Name of the Child: Health and Welfare, 1880–1940* (London: Routledge, 1992); Veronica Strong-Boag and Cheryl Krasnick Warsh, eds., *Children's Health Issues in Historical Perspective* (Waterloo: Wilfrid Laurier University, 2005); Marijke Gijswijt-Hofstra and Hilary Marland, eds., *Cultures of Child Health in Britain and the Netherlands in the Twentieth Century* (Amsterdam and New York: Rodopi, 2003).

11 See, for example, Sydney A. Halpern, *American Pediatrics: The Social Dynamics of Professionalism, 1880–1980* (Berkeley: University of California Press, 1988); Charles R. King, *Children's Health in America: A History* (New York: Twayne Publishers, 1993); Heather Prescott Munro, *A Doctor of Their Own: The History of Adolescent Medicine* (Cambridge, MA: Harvard University Press, 1998). Heather Prescott Munro's history of the development of adolescent medicine in the United States is particularly noteworthy. Concerned primarily with explaining the emergence of this medical sub-specialization in twentieth-century America,

Prescott Munro weaves together issues regarding medical specialization and professionalization, social views regarding adolescence, as well as the concerns and needs of adolescents themselves, and their families.
12 Janet Golden, ed., *Infant Asylums and Children's Hospitals: Medical Dilemmas and Developments, 1850–1920* (New York: Garland, 1989); Judith Young, "'Young Sufferers': Sick Children in Late Nineteenth-Century Toronto," *Nursing History Review* 3 (1995): 129–42; Annmarie Adams and David Theodore, "The Architecture of Children's Hospitals in Toronto and Montreal, 1875–2010," in Veronica Strong-Boag and Cheryl Krasnick Warsh, eds., *Children's Health Issues in Historical Perspective* (Waterloo: Wilfrid Laurier University, 2005), 439–78.
13 See Tony Gould, *A Summer Plague: Polio and its Survivors* (New Haven, CT: Yale University Press, 1995); Christopher Rutty, "The Middle-Class Plague: Epidemic Polio and the Canadian State, 1936–1937," *Canadian Bulletin of Medical History* 13, 2 (1996): 277–314; Janet Golden, *Message in a Bottle: The Making of Fetal Alcohol Syndrome* (Cambridge, MA: Harvard University Press, 2005); John Christopher Feudtner, *Bittersweet: Diabetes, Insulin, and the Transformation of Illness* (Chapel Hill: University of North Carolina Press, 2003).
14 Esyllt Jones, *Influenza 1918: Death, Disease, and Struggle in Winnipeg* (Toronto: University of Toronto Press, 2007). My discussion of the experience of Marc Trapier in chapter 2 of this study includes his childhood experience of growing up in Montreal in the midst of the 1918 influenza in the early decades of the twentieth century.
15 Denise Gastaldo, "Is health education good for you? Rethinking health education through the concept of bio-power," in Alan Peterson and Robin Bunton, eds., *Foucault, Health, and Medicine* (London and New York: Routledge, 1997), 113.
16 Robert McIntosh, "Constructing the Child: New Approaches to the History of Childhood in Canada," *Acadiensis* 18, 2 (Spring 1999): 126–40. For a useful overview in the American context, see Charles R. King, *Children's Health in America: A History*.
17 Patricia T. Rooke and R.L. Schnell, *Discarding the Asylum: From Child Rescue to the Welfare State 1880–1950* (Lanham, MD: University Press of America, 1983).
18 Hugh Cunningham, "Introduction," *Children and Childhood in Western Society Since 1500*, 2nd Edition (Harlow: Pearson Longman, 2005), 1–17.
19 Ibid.; Veronica Strong-Boag, "Getting to Now: Children in Distress in Canada's Past," 31–6.
20 Zelizer, *Pricing the Priceless Child*.

21 On the establishment of physical and sexual "norms" for Canadian adolescents in advice literature in the late nineteenth and early twentieth centuries, see Jennifer Susan Marotta, "Constructing the Norm: Medical Advice Literature to Canadian Adolescents, c. 1873–1922," unpublished Master's thesis, Department of History, Queen's University, 1998.

22 Roger Cooter, ed., *In the Name of the Child – Health and Welfare, 1880–1940* (London and New York: Routledge, 1992); Stern and Markel, *Formative Years*; Marijke Gijswijt-Hofstra and Hilary Marland, eds., *Cultures of Child Health in Britain and the Netherlands in the Twentieth Century* (Amsterdam and New York: Rodopi, 2003); Strong-Boag and Warsh, *Children's Health Issues in Historical Perspective*; Mona Gleason, Tamara Myers, Leslie Paris, and Veronica Strong-Boag, *Lost Kids: Vulnerable Children and Youth in Twentieth-Century Canada and the United States* (Vancouver: UBC Press, 2010); Comacchio, *Nations are Built of Babies*. Comacchio's study of state-sponsored efforts to improve the health and welfare of Ontario's mothers and babies makes similar claims. She concludes that the while infant and maternal mortality rates improved in the period between 1900 and 1940, medical authority was given heightened social status, typically over and above the opinions or desires of families.

23 Nic Clarke, "Sacred Daemons: Exploring British Columbian Society's Perceptions of 'Mentally Deficient' Children, 1870–1930," *BC Studies* 144 (Winter 04/05): 61–90.

24 Charles E. Bourgeois (translated by Paul E. Marquis), *The Protection of Children in the Province of Quebec* (Trois-Rivieres: M. Roy, 1948), 21–2.

25 Baillargeon, *Babies for the Nation*, 183–5.

26 Cynthia Comacchio, *The Dominion of Youth: Adolescence and the Making of Modern Canada, 1920–1950* (Waterloo: Wilfrid Laurier University Press, 2006).

27 Robert McIntosh, "'Grotesque Faces and Figures': Child Labourers and Coal Mining Technology in Victorian Canada," *Scientia Canadensis* 12, 2 (Fall/Winter 1988): 97–112; Robert McIntosh, *Boys in the Pit: Child Labour in Coal Mines* (Montreal & Kingston: McGill-Queen's University Press, 2000).

28 Katherine Arnup, "'Victims of Vaccination?': Opposition to Compulsory Immunization in Ontario, 1900–90," *Canadian Bulletin of Medical History* 9 (1992): 159–76; Gleason, "Race, Class, and Health"; Tamara Myers, "Embodying Delinquency: Boys' Bodies, Sexuality, and Juvenile Justice History in Early Twentieth-Century Quebec," *Journal of the History of Sexuality* 14, 4 (October, 2005): 383–414; Catherine Carstairs

and Rachel Elder, "Expertise, Health, and Popular Opinion: Debating Water Fluoridation, 1945–1980," *Canadian Historical Review* 89, 3 (September, 2008): 345–71.

29 The provision of compulsory public schooling for children spread across the country just prior to the period under study, starting with Ontario by the mid-nineteenth century, Nova Scotia in 1874, the Northwest Territories in 1901, and Alberta and Saskatchewan in 1905. On the history of schooling legislation in Canada, see J.D. Wilson, Robert M. Stamp, and Louis-Phillippe Audet, *Canadian Education – A History* (Scarborough: Prentice Hall of Canada, Ltd., 1970); F. Henry Johnson, *A Brief History of Canadian Education* (Toronto: McGraw-Hill, 1968). In 1943, Quebec enacted the *Compulsory School Attendance Act* under Premier Abélard Godbout. Marshall, *Social Origins of the Welfare State*, 2.

30 Agnes Deans Cameron, "Parent and Teacher," *Canadian Magazine of Politics, Science, Art and Literature* XV (May-October, 1900), 538.

31 On the production of health curriculum priorities in English Canada over the twentieth century and their meaning for children and families, see Gleason, "Between Education and Memory," 49–72.

32 School medical inspections revealed this contradictory aspect of schooling for health in unhealthy schools early in the twentieth century in British Columbia, for example. See Gleason, "Race, Class, and Health."

33 For a discussion of infant mortality as invented, see David Armstrong, "The Invention of Infant Mortality," *Sociology of Health and Illness* 8 (1986): 211–32; H.A. Ansley, "State of Health of People of Canada, 1945," *Canadian Journal of Public Health* 38, 6 (June 1947), 273. By the 1920s, 102 infants per thousand live births died. In 1931, eighty-five out of every thousand infants died. By 1941, the rate dropped to sixty and by 1945, the rate of infant death had declined further to fifty-one out of every thousand live births.

34 C. Collins-Williams, "Accidents in Children," *Canadian Medical Association Journal* 65, 6 (December, 1951): 534.

35 Antonia S. Stang and Arvind Joshi, "The Evolution of Freestanding Children's Hospitals in Canada," *Paediatric Child Health* 11, 8 (October, 2006): 502.

36 Ibid.

37 Canadian Mental Health Association, "Suicide Statistics." *http://www.ontario.cmha.ca/fact_sheets.asp?cID=3965* (Retrieved February 5, 2012).

38 Sutherland, *Children in English-Canadian Society*.

39 Minnett and Poutanen, "Swatting Flies for Health."

40 Stang and Joshi, "The Evolution of Freestanding Children's Hospitals in Canada," 502.

41 Janice Hill, "Politicizing Canadian Childhood Using a Governmentality Framework," *Histoire sociale/Social History* 33, 65 (2000), 176.
42 Wendy Mitchinson, *The Nature of Their Bodies – Women and Their Doctors in Victorian Canada* (Toronto: University of Toronto Press, 1991); *Giving Birth in Canada: 1900 to 1950* (Toronto: University of Toronto, 2002).
43 Marshall, *The Social Origins of the Welfare State*, x–xi.
44 In the context of Canada, both Tamara Myers and Cynthia Comacchio have demonstrated that the rise of adolescence as a separate, biological stage in the life course and a socio-historical construction over the course of the twentieth century marks a distinctive historical process. Tamara Myers, *Caught: Montreal's Modern Girls and the Law, 1869–1945* (Toronto: University of Toronto Press, 2006); Comacchio, *The Dominion of Youth*. Jennifer Susan Marotta has studied the role of medical advice literature in constructing "norms" of embodiment and behaviour in Canadian adolescence over the turn of the twentieth century. Jennifer Susan Marotta, "Constructing the Norm: Medical Advice Literature to Canadian Adolescents, c. 1873–1922," unpublished Master's thesis, Queen's University, 1998.
45 An important recent collection that takes up the meanings attached to children's embodiment in contemporary society is Kathrin Hörschelmann and Rachel Colls, *Contested Bodies of Childhood and Youth* (Hampshire: Palgrave McMillan, 2010).
46 Joan Wallace Scott, "Gender as a Useful Category of Historical Analysis," *American Historical Review* 91, 5 (December, 1986): 1053–76.
47 As *linked* theoretical concepts, age and size are not well-developed in historical scholarship devoted to children and youth. Age, however, has attracted scholarly attention. See, for example, the forum discussion in the inaugural volume of *Journal of the History of Childhood and Youth* 1, 1 (Winter, 2008): 89–156. Age and age-consciousness as *subjects* of historical inquiry have commanded the attention of scholars such as Howard Chudacoff. Chudacoff found that age-consciousness and age-grading developed at the turn of the twentieth century in the American context, largely the result of shifts in education and medicine, was "adopted as an organizing principle reflecting people's need for ordering and understanding modern life." Howard P. Chudacoff, *How Old are You? Age Consciousness in American Culture* (New Jersey: Princeton University Press, 1989).
48 David Michael Levin and George F. Solomon, "The Discursive Formation of the Body in the History of Medicine," *The Journal of Medicine and Philosophy* 15 (1990): 515–16.
49 Barrie Thorne, "Editorial: Crafting the Interdisciplinary field of Childhood Studies," *Childhood* 14, 2 (May 2007): 149–50. Thinking about and

treating children as "potentialities rather than actualities," in Claudia Castaneda's phrase, has dominated both discursive representations of children and material aspects of adult-child relations in the West for centuries. Claudia Castaneda, *Figuration: Child, Bodies, Worlds* (Durham and London: Duke University Press, 2002), 1.

50 The interviews used in this book were selected from a larger pool of sixty-two interviews (interviews are labeled as the Child Health Project for the purposes of this book). Participants were encouraged to talk about what they remembered about health and illness in their childhoods. Attempts were made in this book to choose interviews with women and men from a wide variety of backgrounds. Those oral history interviews used here include adults who grew up in western, central, and eastern Canada, from working-class, lower-middle, and middle-class, and from Anglo-Celtic, Anglo-Saxon, Asian, and First Nation backgrounds. The interviewees were selected primarily through word of mouth and some limited advertising in retirement homes in Vancouver, Penticton, and Montreal. We relied primarily on a snowball effect in which those interviewed told friends and family who in turn contacted us. The interview questions were intentionally broad and asked participants for their childhood recollections of anything to do with health, health care, learning to be healthy, illness, and medical treatment. We asked only that participants be raised in Canada and born before 1960.

51 Sutherland, *Growing Up*, 3–23. I address the utility of oral histories and autobiographies in Gleason, "Disciplining the Student Body" and Gleason, "Embodied Negotiations." See also, Paul Thompson, "Believe it or No: Rethinking the Historical Interpretation of Memory," in Jaclyn Jeffrey and Glenace Edwall, eds., *Memory and History: Essays on Recalling and Interpreting Experience* (Lanham, New York: University Press of American, 1994), 6–7. On the problems and potentials associated with autobiography as a historical source, see Sutherland, *Growing Up*; John Sturrock, *The Language of Autobiography – Studies in the First Person Singular* (London: Cambridge University Press, 1993), 1–19; Richard Coe, *When the Grass was Taller – Autobiography and the Experience of Childhood* (New Haven: Yale University Press, 1984).

52 George Morgan, "Unsettling Narratives," in *Unsettled Places – Aboriginal People and Urbanisation in New South Wales* (Kent Town: Wakefield Press, 2006), 107. I am indebted to Dr Kalervo Gulson for bringing my attention to this work.

53 Ian Hacking, "Making Up People," in Thomas C. Heller, Morton Sasna, and David E. Wellbery, eds., *Reconstructing Individualism: Autonomy,*

Individuality, and the Self in Western Thought (California: Stanford University Press, 1986), 223.

54 All names have changed to protect the anonymity of interviewees.

55 Most recently, Denyse Baillargeon has offered an important groundbreaking study of programs aimed at hospitalized children in "Learning and Leisure on the Inside: Programs for Children at Sainte-Justine Hospital, 1925–70," in Gleason et al., *Lost Kids*, 117–35.

56 Although this study does not focus exclusively on the history of children with disabilities, I attempt here to take up Richard J. Altenbaugh's most recent call for historians to pay more critical attention to the question: "What impact does disability in general and disease in particular have on childhood?" (719). Richard J. Altenbaugh, "Where are the Disabled in the History of Education? The Impact of Polio on Sites of Learning," *History of Education* 35, 6 (November, 2006): 705–30.

CHAPTER ONE

1 See, for example, Minnett and Poutanen "Swatting Flies for Health."

2 Wendy Mitchinson, *The Nature of Their Bodies – Women and Their Doctors in Victorian Canada* (Toronto: University of Toronto Press, 1991); Wendy Mitchinson, *Giving Birth in Canada, 1900–1950* (Toronto: University of Toronto, 2002).

3 Michel Foucault, "The Subject and Power," *Critical Inquiry* 8, 4 (Summer, 1982): 777–95. Ian Hacking makes a similar point: "Social change creates new categories of people, but the counting is no mere report of developments. It elaborately, often philanthropically, creates new ways for people to be." Ian Hacking, "Making Up People," in Thomas C. Heller, Morton Sosna, and David E. Wellbery, eds., *Reconstructing Individualism: Autonomy, Individuality, and the Self in Western Thought* (Stanford: Stanford University Press, 1986), 222–36.

4 A.R. Colón with P.A. Colón, *Nuturing Children – A History of Pediatrics* (Westport, Ct: Greenwood Press, 1999), x–xvi.

5 Jacalyn Duffy, "No Baby, No Nation: A History of Pediatrics," in *History of Medicine – A Scandalously Short Introduction* (Toronto: University of Toronto Press, 1999), 303; Colón with Colón, *Nuturing Children*, xiv; Angel Ballabriga, "One Century of Pediatrics in Europe," in Buford L. Nichols, Angel Ballabriga, and Norman Kretchmer, eds., *History of Pediatrics, 1850–1950* (New York: Raven Press, 1991), 2.

6 See, for example, Rene Norcross, "The Little Brother," *The Canadian Nurse*, II (1915): 436–38; Robert Bell, *The "Medicine-Man", or, Indian*

and Eskimo Notions of Medicine (Montreal: Gazette Printing Company, 1886); Kathleen Stewart, "At Work in an Indian School," *Canadian Nurse* 38, 2 (February, 1942): 115–16.
7 Pye Henry Chavasse, *Advice to a Mother on the Management of Her Children and on the Treatment on the Moment of Some of Their More Pressing Illnesses and Accidents* (Toronto: Willing and Williamson, 1880), 2. Chavasse quotes from "Dr W. Lindsay Alexander, Good Words, March, 1861."
8 On the increasing professional dominance over matters of children's health in the early decades of the twentieth century, see Anonymous, "The Health of the Child," *Canadian Medical Association Journal* 2, 8 (August 1912): 704–5; J. Halpenny and Lillian Ireland, *How to be Healthy* (Winnipeg and Toronto: W.J. Gage and Company, 1911), 174; C.A. Lucas, *Public Health Education in the Schools* (British Columbia: Provincial Board of Health, 1926), 3; John W.S. McCullough, "Are you Sure of Their Health? An Interesting Challenge to Parents and Teachers Everywhere," *Chatelaine* (December, 1930): 9, 57.
9 W.J. Stevens, "A Review of Obstetrics," *Canadian Nurse* 23, 9 (September, 1927): 465. Summarizing the importance of routine and structure in "modern" child-rearing, professional child-rearing advice to mothers called upon them to treat their babies like "little machines." See Lewis, "Creating the Little Machine."
10 Adams and Theodore, "Children's Hospitals in Toronto and Montreal"; Young, "'Little Sufferers'," 130.
11 Ibid. In 1885 a clinic for children was established under the auspices of Les Dormes de la Charité de la Providence in Quebec City. The Montreal Foundling and Baby Hospital appeared in 1892 (later amalgamated into the Children's Memorial Hospital); the Hospital for Sick Children in Toronto in 1875; the Winnipeg Children's Hospital opened in 1909; Halifax Children's Hospital appeared in 1910; the War Memorial Children's Hospital opened in London, Ontario in 1922. Pediatric admissions to general hospitals, such as the Kingston General Hospital in Kingston, Ontario, occurred in the late 1800s.
12 J.B.J. McKendry and J.D. Bailey, *Paediatrics in Canada* (Ottawa: Canadian Paediatric Society, 1990), 4–5.
13 Ibid., 4–11. In 1905, pediatrics became a separate specialization from obstetrics at the Faculty of Medicine at Queen's University. In 1933, Dr Michael Carney, became the first professor of pediatrics at Dalhousie University's medical school. The Pediatric Department at the University of Manitoba emerged in the 1920s; 1919 at the University of Alberta.

14 Howard Markel, "For the Welfare of Children" in Stern and Markel, *Formative Years*, 48.
15 Nichols, et. al., *History of Pediatrics, 1850–1950* (New York: Raven Press, 1991); see particularly Buford L. Nichols Jr., "The European Roots of American Pediatrics," 49–54; Howard A. Pearson, "Pediatrics in the United States," 55–64; Silvestre Frenk and Ignacio Avila-Cisneros, "Mexican Pediatrics," 65–76. On the connections made between public health and pediatrics see, for example, "Chapter 13: No Baby, No Nation: A History of Pediatrics," in Duffin, *History of Medicine*; George Weisz, *Divide and Conquer – A Comparative History of Medical Specialization* (Toronto: Oxford University Press, 2006); Russell Viner, "Abraham Jacobi and the Origins of Scientific Pediatrics in America," in Stern and Markel, *Formative Years*, 23–46.
16 On the difference class made to infant mortality rates, see Comacchio, *Nations Are Built of Babies*, especially "Chapter 2: 'Guarded Against Harmful Conditions': The Campaign's Setting," 16–42; on the role of racism and First Nation vulnerability, see Tina Moffat and Ann Herring, "The Historical Roots of High Rates of Infant Death in Aboriginal Communities in Canada in the early twentieth century: the case of Fisher River, Manitoba," *Social Science and Medicine* 48 (1999), 1821–32.
17 Mary Anne Poutanen points out that this rate of death from tuberculosis was likely higher given that deaths from diseases listed as pneumonia, meningitis, and other deadly childhood afflictions, were likely more accurately the result of tuberculosis. Mary Anne Poutanen, "Containing and Preventing Contagious Disease: Montreal's Protestant School Board and Tuberculosis, 1900–1947," *Canadian Bulletin of Medical History* 23, 2 (2006): 404.
18 Moffat and Herring, "The Historical Roots of High Rates of Infant Deaths in Aboriginal Communities in Canada."
19 Sutherland, *Children in English-Canadian Society*, 57.
20 As quoted in Nora Moore, "Child Welfare Work," *The Canadian Nurse* 12, 11 (November, 1916): 634–5.
21 Comacchio, *Nations Are Built of Babies*, especially "Chapter 2: 'Guarded Against Harmful Conditions': The Campaign's Setting," 16–42.
22 As quoted in Moore, "Child Welfare Work," 634.
23 Minnett and Poutanen, "Swatting Flies for Health"; Comacchio, *Nations Are Built of Babies*, 16–42; Sutherland, *Children in English-Canadian Society*, especially Part II: "'To Create A Strong and Healthy Race' – Children in the Public Health Movement, 1880–1920," 39–79.

24 Anonymous, "Health Centre Work a Living Memorial," (*Victoria Daily Times* August 21, 1919): 18.
25 Sutherland, *Children in English-Canadian Society*; Comacchio, *Nations Are Built of Babies*.
26 Ernest Couture, "Some Aspects of the Child Health Program in Canada," *Canadian Public Health Journal* 30, 12 (December 1939): 580–4; L. Emmett Holt, "Health Education of Children," *Canadian Public Health Journal* 13, 3 (March 1922): 106.
27 Holt, "Health Education of Children," 106.
28 On the eugenics movement in Canada, see Angus MacLaren, *Our Own Master Race: Eugenics in Canada, 1885–1945* (Toronto: University of Toronto Press, 1990). See also Comacchio, *Nations are Built of Babies*, 18–20; Sharon L. Snyder and David T. Mitchell, *Cultural Locations of Disability* (Chicago and London: The University of Chicago Press, 2006), ix.
29 Henry Ashby and G.A. Wright, *The Diseases of Children – Medical and Surgical* (New York: Longmans, Green and Co., Medical Publishers, 1897), 1. This text was distributed in Canada by A.P. Watts & Co., "Medical Publishers and Booksellers to College St., Toronto."
30 D.J. Dunn, "Medical Inspection of School Children," *Canadian Medical Association Journal* 8, 10 (October, 1918): 926, 932.
31 Couture, "Some Aspects of the Child Health Program in Canada."
32 Stang and Joshi, "The Evolution of Freestanding Children's Hospitals in Canada," 502.
33 Statistics Canada, Historical Statistics, "Series B59–64. Average Annual Infant Death Rates for Selected Causes, Canada, for Five Year Periods, 1931 to 1974." http://www.statcan.gc.ca/pub/11-516-x/sectionb/4147437-eng.htm#1 (Retrieved 17 February 2012).
34 Kenneth N. Fenwick, *Manual of Obstetrics, Gynaecology, and Pediatrics* (Kingston: J. Henderson, 1889), 192. Fenwick was a professor of obstetrics and diseases of women and children at the Royal College of Physicians and Surgeons and an affiliate of Queen's University in Kingston, Ontario.
35 Ashby and Wright, *The Diseases of Children*, 2–3.
36 Ibid.
37 George E. Smith, "The Prevention of Infection in Infancy," *The Public Health Journal* 17, 8 (August 1926), 405–6.
38 Hector Charles Campbell, *Diseases of Childhood – A Short Introduction* (London: Oxford University Press, 1926), 6–7. This text was utilized by teaching staff at the University of British Columbia's Faculty of Medicine.

39 Ibid.
40 Hector Charles Cameron, "Sleep and its Disorders in Childhood," *Canadian Medical Association Journal* 24, 2 (February 1931): 241.
41 Ibid.
42 Lewis, "Creating the Little Machine," 51–2.
43 Fenwick, *Manual of Obstetrics, Gynaecology, and Pediatrics*, 193.
44 Alan Brown and Frederick F. Tisdall, *Common Procedures in the Practice of Paediatrics*, 4th ed. (Toronto: McClelland and Stewart, 1949), 7. The first edition of the work appeared in 1929. The fourth edition was revised to reflect the arrival of sulpha drugs and to reflect "a better understanding of the fundamental principles of mineral metabolism" (preface to fourth edition).
45 Ibid.
46 O.M. Moore, "Peptic Ulcers in Children," *Canadian Medical Association Journal* 44, 5 (May, 1941): 462–6.
47 Alan Brown, "Some Factors Concerning the Care of the Newborn," *Canadian Public Health Journal* 29, 7 (July 1938): 339.
48 "Kleenex (Advertisement)," *Chatelaine* (March, 1936): 62. See also "Vicks VapoRub (Advertisement)," *Chatelaine* (March, 1936): 61; Zam-Buk (Advertisement), *Victoria Daily Times* October 31, 1919, 6.
49 Lloyd P. MacHaffie, "Pitfalls and Tragedies of the Pre-School Child," *Child and Family Welfare* 12, 1 (May 1936): 11.
50 Nelles Silverthorne, "Meningitis in Childhood," *Canadian Medical Association Journal* 48, 3 (March 1943): 218.
51 Olive B. Warren, "Rheumatic Fever: Scourge of Childhood," *The Canadian Nurse* 45, 11 (1949): 857.
52 Chavasse, *Advice to a Mother on the Management of her Children*, 263.
53 William Briggs, *Manual of Hygiene for Schools and Colleges* (Toronto: Provincial Board of Health, 1886), 140.
54 Ibid., 141.
55 For more sustained analysis on the role of health curriculum in the construction of healthy children see especially "Chapter 4: Learning the Body: Schools, Curriculum, and Health."
56 William Krohn, *First Book in Hygiene – A Primer in Physiology* (New York: D. Appleton and Company, 1907), 122.
57 Charles H. Stowell, *The Essentials of Health. A Text-book on Anatomy, Physiology, and Hygiene* (Toronto: The Educational Book Company, Ltd., 1909), 15.
58 William Krohn, *First Book in Hygiene*, 120–3.

59 Nora Moore, "Child Welfare Work," *The Canadian Nurse* 12, 11 (November 1916): 633.
60 J. Wyllie, "Sex Differences in the Mortalities of Childhood and Adult Life," *Canadian Public Health Journal* 24, 11 (Nov. 1933): 530–42.
61 E.W. McHenry, "Nutrition and Child Health," *Canadian Public Health Journal* 33, 4 (April 1942): 54.
62 Helen Boyd, "Growing Up Privileged in Edmonton," *Alberta History* 30, 1 (1982): 4–5.
63 Annabelle Lee, "Beauty," *Chatelaine* (September, 1932): 26.
64 Moore, "Child Welfare Work," 634.
65 Tamara Myers, "From Disciplinarian to Coach: The Policing of Youth in Mid-20th Century Canada," (Unpublished) paper presented to European Social Science History Association Conference, Lisbon, 26 February to 1 March 2008. In this paper, Myers traces the establishment of the Montreal police service's Juvenile Morality Squad (JMS) in 1936. The JMS "explored the causes of juvenile delinquency by looking at the role played by adults in promoting adolescent immorality. It was under Articles 29 and 33 of the *Juvenile Delinquents Act* (Canada, 1908) that the juvenile court held jurisdiction over adults who were deemed responsible for juvenile delinquency. Under these articles the juvenile court processed several hundred adults each year." See also Myers, *Caught: Montreal's Modern Girls and the Law, 1869–1945*, 195, on the ineffectual use of Articles 29 and 33 to protect children from incest.
66 Moore, "Child Welfare Work," 635.
67 B.E.A. Philmot, "In the Children's Ward," *The Canadian Nurse* 5 (1910): 176–7. Myra Rutherdale explores similar process of "cleaning" Aboriginal children in "Ordering the Bath: Children, Health and Hygiene in Northern Communities, 1900–1970," in Strong-Boag and Warsh, *Children's Health Issues in Historical Perspective*, 305–24.
68 Ibid., 176.
69 Library and Archives Canada (LAC), MG 28 I 343, Canadian Medical Association (CMA), Volume 7, File 1, Minutes (book) CMA Section of Public Health, "Report of the Pediatric Section of the CMA, 18 June 1924, 73.
70 A. Grant Fleming, "The Value of Periodic Health Examinations," *The Canadian Nurse* 25, 6 (June 1929): 284.
71 L. Emmett Holt, "Health Education of Children," *Canadian Public Health Journal* 13, 3 (March 1922): 113.
72 As quoted in Moffatt and Herring, "The Historical Roots of High Rates of Infant Death," 1829.

73 Ibid., 1828.
74 Florence C. Moffat, "Forgotten Villages of the BC Coast – Hospital Life at Bella Bella," *Raincoast Chronicles* 11 (1987): 52.
75 Margery Hind, *School House in the Arctic* (London: Geoffrey Bles, 1958), 95.
76 R.P Vivian, Charles McMillan, P.E. Moore, E. Chant Robertson, W.H Sebrell, F.F. Tisdall, and W.G. McIntosh, "The Nutrition and Health of the James Bay Indian," *Canadian Medical Association Journal* 59, 6 (December, 1948), 505.
77 See Kelm, *Colonizing Bodies*.
78 Numerous accounts of residential school life in Canada bring up the issue of lack of adequate food. See, for example, Basil Johnston, *Indian School Days* (Toronto: Key Porter Books, 1988); Sylvia Olsen, *No Time to Say Goodbye: Children's Stories of Kuper Island Residential School* (Victoria: Sono Nis Press, 2001); Shirley Sterling, *My Name is Seepeetza* (Toronto: Douglas and McIntyre, 1992).

CHAPTER TWO

1 Comacchio, *Nations are Built of Babies*, 3–6.
2 Desmond Morton, "Military Medicine and State Medicine: Historical Notes on the Canadian Army Corps in the First World War, 1914–1919," in C. David Naylor, ed., *Canadian Health Care and the State – A Century of Evolution* (Montreal & Kingston: McGill-Queen's University Press, 1992), 38–66.
3 All proper names are pseudonyms.
4 Christopher J. Rutty, "The Twentieth Century Plague," *The Beaver* 84, 2 (April/May 2004): 32–7.
5 Ibid.
6 Child Health Project (CHP), Interview 23, transcript, 1.
7 Ibid., 1–2.
8 Sidney Herman Licht, "History of Electrotherapy", in Sidney Licht, ed., *Therapeutic Electricity and Ultraviolet Radiation*, 2nd edition. (New Haven: E. Licht, 1967), 1–70.
9 The evolution of a publicly funded system began in the prairie province of Saskatchewan in 1946. In that year, Premier Tommy Douglas's Co-operative Commonwealth Federation government passed the *Saskatchewan Hospitalization Act* which gave much of the population free hospital care. By the 1960s, similar acts and the extension of more comprehensive benefits were in place across the country. C. David Naylor,

rivate Practice, Public Payment: Canadian Medicine and the Politics of Health Insurance 1911–1966 (Montreal & Kingston: McGill-Queen's University Press, 1986).

10 CHP, Interview 23, transcript, 7.
11 CHP, Interview 17, transcript, 5.
12 I am grateful to Molly Ladd-Taylor who suggested this phrase to signify young people's ability to exercise control in their lives. For an incorporation of this concept in an earlier study, see Gleason, "Lost Voices, Lost Bodies?" in Gleason et al., *Lost Kids*, 136–53.
13 See chapter 5 in this study. Denyse Baillargeon has offered a very useful analysis of attempts to address the needs of children in one Montreal hospital in "Learning and Leisure on the Inside: Programs for Sick Children at Sainte-Justine Hospital, 1925–1970," in Gleason et al., *Lost Kids*, 117–35.
14 M.W. Partington, "Paediatric Admissions to Kingston General Hospital, Kingston Ontario (1899–1909)," *Families* 22, 1 (1983): 33–46. Mother and child admissions accounted for 13 per cent of pediatric cases over the period under study.
15 CHP, Interview 23, transcript, 9.
16 Ibid.
17 For a fuller treatment of attitudes towards children and disability in this period see chapter 6 in this study.
18 CHP, Interview 23, transcript, 7.
19 Ibid., transcript, 11.
20 Ibid.
21 Sources that discuss the unsuitability of non-professional medical practices and practitioners included William Briggs, *Manual of Hygiene for Schools and Colleges* (Toronto: Provincial Board of Health, 1886), 9; J.W.S. McCullough, "Chatelaine's Baby Clinic: The Common Diseases," *Chatelaine* 6 (1934): 54; J. Mace Andress and Elizabeth Breeze, *Health Essentials for Canadian Schools* (Boston, Montreal, and London: Ginn, 1938), 159; Ross A. Campbell, "The Spastic Child," *Canadian Nurse* 42 (1946): 471.
22 CHP, Interview 24, transcript, 1.
23 Jacques Ferland, "In Search of the Unbound Prometheia: A Comparative View of Women's Activism in Two Quebec Industries, 1869–1908," *Labour/ Le Travail* 24 (Spring 1989): 11–44. On 14 April 1880, women in the Hochelaga mill instigated the first work stoppage recorded for the cotton industry.
24 CHP, Interview 24, transcript, 2.
25 Ibid., transcript, 9.

26 Ibid.
27 Mary Anne Poutanen, "Containing and Preventing Contagious Disease: Montreal's Protestant School Board and Tuberculosis," *Canadian Bulletin of Medical History* 23, 2 (2006): 403–5.
28 CHP, Interview 24, transcript, 9.
29 Ibid.
30 See Esyllt Jones for Winnipeg's experience with the 1918 flu pandemic and its toll on family life in *Influenza, 1918: Disease, Death, and Struggle in Winnipeg* (Toronto: University of Toronto Press, 2007).
31 CHP, Interview 24, transcript, 5.
32 On the use of coal oil as a popular remedy see Austin E. Fife, "Popular Legends of the Mormons," *California Folklore Quarterly* 1, 2 (April, 1942): 105–25.
33 CHP, Interview 24, transcript, 6.
34 Esyllt Jones, *Influenza 1918*, "Chapter 7: Family Life after Influenza: Single Parents and Orphans," 141–64.
35 CHP, Interview 24, transcript, 7.
36 Ibid.
37 Poutanen, "Containing and Preventing Contagious Disease," 404.
38 CHP, Interview 5, transcript, 2.
39 Ibid., 2.
40 Ibid.
41 Ibid.
42 On early twentieth-century opposition see Katherine Arnup, "'Victims of Vaccination'?: Opposition to Compulsory Immunization in Ontario, 1900–1990," *Canadian Bulletin of Medical History* 9 (1992): 159–76.
43 CHP, Interview 5, transcript, 3.
44 Ibid., 4.
45 Ibid.
46 Ashby and Wright, *The Diseases of Children*, 56–7; Jean Browne, "School Nursing in Regina," *Canadian Nurse* 7, 9 (September, 1911): 439–45; Moore, "Child Welfare Work," 634–35; L. Emmett Holt, "Health Education of Children," *Canadian Public Health Journal*, 13, 3 (March 1922): 106–13.
47 Moore, "Child Welfare Work," 588.
48 Janie Dearland had a typical experience. Janie grew up in Saskatoon in the 1930s and had her teeth filled by a dentist who came to her public school: "And he drilled, I mean there were no painkillers injected into my gums, and I can remember I was terrified, and from that day on I was terrified and I just didn't like going to the dentist, and I think that you'll find

a lot of us our age are terrified of the dentist and won't go, and I think you'll find that a lot of us put off going because we had that first experience." CHP, Interview 18N, transcript, 10.
49 CHP, Interview 5, transcript, 7.
50 Ibid., 3.
51 Ibid., 10.
52 CHP, Interview 10, transcript 2.
53 Ibid., 2.
54 Florence P. Kendall, "Sister Kenny Revisited," *Archives of Physical Medicine and Rehabilitation* 79, 4 (1998): 361–5; Victor Cohn, *Sister Kenny: The Woman Who Challenged the Doctors* (Burns and MacEachern Limited: Don Mills, 1975).
55 CHP, Interview 10, transcript 3.
56 Ibid.
57 Ibid., 7.
58 Ibid., 8.
59 See also the quarantine experience of Amelia Desjardin in the conclusion of this book.
60 CHP, Interview 10, transcript 10.
61 Ibid., 5.
62 Ibid.
63 Ibid., 4.
64 Ibid., 9.
65 Ibid., 5.
66 Ibid., 7.
67 Jean Browne, "School Nursing in Regina," *Canadian Nurse* VII, 9 (September, 1911): 449.
68 A typical example is C.J. Fagan, "Contagious Disease," in Charles H. Stowell, *The Essentials of Health. A Text-book on Anatomy, Physiology, and Hygiene.* The New Health Series of School Physiologies (Toronto: The Educational Book Company, Ltd. Toronto. 1909), 286.
69 CHP, Interview 23, transcript, 12.

CHAPTER THREE

1 Although the Canadian infant mortality rate fell from an average of eighty deaths to an average of seventy-one deaths (per thousand live births) between 1930 and 1940, many professionals at the time considered it still unacceptably high. See chapter 1. Statistics Canada (2008-10-22). "Series

B23–34. Average Age Specific Death-Rates, Both Sexes. Canada for five-year periods, 1921–1974." *http://www.statcan.gc.ca/pub/11-516-x/ sectionb/4147437-eng.htm* (Retrieved on 25 March 2010)

2 Epidemics of small pox were constant features of life in Canada. Montreal suffered a major small pox epidemic in late 1880s, while Windsor was struck in 1924. Between 1929 and 1933, there were 4548 cases and thirty-six deaths. The Indigenous small pox cases in Canada were recorded in 1945–56 with seven cases in Saskatchewan. On the history of small pox and its containment in Canada see Luis Bareto and Christopher Rutty, "The Speckled Monster: Canada, Small pox, and its Eradication" *Canadian Journal of Public Health* 93, 4 (2002): 12–30.

3 On controversy over water fluoridation, see P.R. Crawford, "Fifty Years of Fluoridation"; Catherine Carstairs and Rachel Elder, "Expertise, Health and Popular Opinion."

4 University of Toronto, "History of the Department of Paediatrics – Historical Perspectives." *http://www.paeds.utoronto.ca/about/history.htm* (Retrieved 25 March 2010)

5 Gleason, "Race, Class, and Health."

6 Andress and Breeze, *Health Essentials for Canadian Schools*, iii.

7 Child Health Project (CHP), Interview 1, transcript, 1.

8 Ibid., 3–4.

9 Ibid., 2.

10 Ibid.

11 Deplorable conditions on many First Nation reserves in Canada continue to be ignored by government. In 2009, Auditor General Sheila Fraser decried the level of environmental pollution on reserves and called on the Federal Government to respond. See Margot McDarmid, "Native reserves polluted due to gaps in rules: AG," CBC News Online, 3 November 2009. *http://www.cbc.ca/canada/story/2009/11/03/vaughan-fraser-auditor-environment-commissioner-report.html* (Retrieved 24 March 2010)

12 CHP, Interview 1, transcript, 2.

13 Ibid., 11.

14 On the silence and misinformation surrounding sexuality in memories of growing up, see Gleason, "Embodied Negotiations." For similar histories in the British context, see Angela Davis, "'Oh, no, nothing, we didn't learn anything': Sex Education and the Preparation of Girls for Motherhood, c. 1930–1970," *History of Education* 37, 5 (September 2008): 661–77; on Australia see Josephine May, "Secrets and Lies: Sex Education and the Gendered Memories of Childhood's End in an Australian Provincial City, 1930s to 1950s," *Sex Education* 6, 1 (February 2006): 1–15. On the

politics of silencing sex education, see Janice M. Irvine, *Talk about Sex: The Battle over Sex Education in the United States* (Berkeley: University of California Press, 2002).
15 CHP, Interview 1, transcript, 13–14.
16 Ibid., 14.
17 Ibid., 14.
18 CHP, Interview 4, transcript, 1.
19 Ibid., 4–5.
20 Ibid., 2.
21 Ibid., 2–3.
22 Ibid., 3.
23 Ibid., 3–4.
24 Ibid., 4.
25 Ibid., 5.
26 See, for example, professional medical calls for the discontinuation of copper sulfate for children in Neil A. Holtzman and Robert Haslam, "Elevation of Serum Copper following Copper Sulfate as an Emetic," *Pediatrics* 42, 1 (July 1968): 189–93; Kent C. Olsen, *Poisoning and Drug Overdose* (New York: Lang Medical Books/McGraw Hill, 2004).
27 CHP, Interview 4, transcript, 10.
28 Ibid., 9.
29 Ibid., 8.
30 Ibid., 12.
31 CHP, Interview 7A, transcript, 1.
32 Ibid., 3.
33 Ibid., 2.
34 Ibid., 3.
35 Ibid., 7.
36 Ibid., 3.
37 Ibid., 10.
38 CHP, Interview 32, transcript, 29N.
39 Ibid., 4.
40 Ibid.
41 Ibid., 6.
42 Christopher Rutty, "The Middle-Class Plague: Epidemic Polio and the Canadian State, 1936–1937," *Canadian Bulletin of Medical History* 13 (1996): 277–314.
43 CHP, Interview 32, transcript, 1.
44 The Queen Alexandra Solarium was opened at Mill Bay on Vancouver Island in 1926. Initiated by the Women's Institutes of British Columbia,

it housed and treated "crippled" children through heliotherapy or the "sun cure."
45 CHP, Interview 32, transcript, 2.
46 Ibid., 2.
47 Ibid., 13.
48 Ibid.
49 J. W. McIntosh, "The Vancouver Outbreak of Haemorrhagic Smallpox II: Lessons Learned from the Outbreak," *Canadian Public Health Journal* 24, 3 (March 1933): 112–19.
50 Robin Jarvis Brownlie, "'Living the Same as White People': Mohawk and Anishinabe Women's Labour in Southern Ontario, 1920–1940," *Labour/ Le Travail* 61 (Spring, 2008), 41–68.

CHAPTER FOUR

1 C.A. Lucas, *Public Health Education in the Schools* (Provincial Board of Health, British Columbia, 1926), 2. A portion of this chapter was first published in Gleason, "Between Education and Memory."
2 Keith Hoskin, "The Examination, Disciplinary Power and Rational Schooling," *History of Education* 8, 2 (1979), 136. See also Daphne Meadmore, "The Production of Individuality through Examination," *British Journal of Sociology of Education* 14, 1 (1993): 59–73.
3 An important exception is Gale Smith and Linda Peterat's work in which they take up the history of health education in Canada briefly in "Reading Between the Lines – Examining Assumptions in Health Education," in Tara Goldstein and David Selby, eds., Weaving *Connections – Educating for Peace, Social and Environmental Justice* (Toronto: Sumach Press, 2000), 242–67.
4 The classic history of curriculum development in Canada is George Tompkins, *A Common Countenance: Stability and Change in the Canadian Curriculum* (Scarborough: Prentice Hall, 1986). Tompkins also makes clear the prominent place of the textbook in school curriculum in Canada at this time.
5 For an interpretation of curriculum as a reflection of social values, see Bernd Baldus and Meenaz Kassam, "'Make me truthful, good and mild': Values in Nineteenth-century Ontario Schoolbooks," *Canadian Journal of Sociology* 21 (1996): 327–58. See also Michael W. Apple and Linda K. Christian-Smith, "The Politics of the Textbook," in Michael W. Apple and Linda K. Christian-Smith, eds., *The Politics of the Textbook* (New York: Routledge, 1991), 1–21.

6 Baldus and Kassam, "Make me truthful, good and mild," 327–8. The textbooks used in the study were produced internally by Canadian authors and publishing houses, and externally, particularly from American sources.
7 Gleason, "Race, Class and Health."
8 The provision of compulsory public schooling for children spread across the country starting with Ontario by the mid-nineteenth century, Manitoba and New Brunswick in 1871, British Columbia in 1872, Newfoundland and Nova Scotia in 1874, the Northwest Territories in 1901, and Alberta and Saskatchewan in 1905. On the history of schooling legislation in Canada, see J.D. Wilson, Robert M. Stamp, and Louis-Phillippe Audet, *Canadian Education – A History* (Scarborough: Prentice-Hall of Canada, Ltd., 1970); F. Henry Johnson, *A Brief History of Canadian Education* (Toronto: McGraw-Hill, 1968). Quebec's compulsory education was introduced in 1943, although the province had a long history of providing for schooling along a dual Catholic and Protestant system. See Marshall, *The Social Origins of the Welfare State*.
9 W.J. Gage, *Gage's Health Series for Intermediate Classes* Part 2 (Toronto: W.J. Gage & Company's Educational Series. Toronto, 1896), 163.
10 On the significance of the temperance movement in Canada see Christie, *Households of Faith*.
11 Knight, *The Ontario Public School Hygiene*, 229.
12 Stowell, *The Essentials of Health*, 253. This text was "prescribed for use in the Public and High Schools of British Columbia," (preface).
13 Wendy Mitchinson, *The Nature of Their Bodies – Women and Their Doctors in Victorian Canada* (Toronto: University of Toronto Press, 1991); Veronica Strong-Boag, *The New Day Recalled – Lives of Girls and Women in English Canada, 1919–1939* (Toronto: Copp Clark Pitman, 1988).
14 J. Halpenny and Lillian Ireland, *How to be Healthy* (Toronto and Winnipeg: W.J. Gage and Company, 1911), 54.
15 See Robert Bell, *The "Medicine Man": or Indian and Eskimo Notions of Medicine* (Montreal: Gazette Printing Company, 1886); Kelm, *Colonizing Bodies*. See also the discussion of the dangers of homespun health practices in J.W.S. McCullough, "Chatelaine's Baby Clinic – The Common Diseases," *Chatelaine*, 6 (1934): 54; Ross A. Campbell, "The Spastic Child," *Canadian Nurse* 42 (1946): 471.
16 From a 1908 report issued by the government of Canada, as cited in Moffat and Herring, "The Historical Roots of High Rates of Infant Death."
17 Kelm, *Colonizing Bodies*.
18 John Dewhirst, "Coast Salish Summer Festivals: Rituals for Upgrading Social Identity," *Anthropologica* 17, 2 (1976): 258.

19 Such rules were repeated in a number of authorized health textbooks. See, for example, William Briggs, *Manual of Hygiene for Schools and Colleges* (Toronto: William Briggs, 1886), 14–5. "Authorized by the Ontario Minister of Education for use in all schools under the control of the Education Department," (preface); Frances Gulick Jewett, *Book One – Good Health (The Gulick Series)* (Boston: Ginn & Company, 1906), 33–5.

20 Knight, *The Ontario Public School Hygiene*, (preface).

21 CHP Interview 7A, transcript, 7. See also the experiences of Florence Drake (chapter 2), Theresa Elliott (chapter 2), and Amelia Desjardin (conclusion).

22 CHP Interview 10N, transcript, 2.

23 CHP Interview 06N, transcript, 6.

24 Ibid.

25 CHP Interview 007N, transcript, 2.

26 This message of the superiority of medical science in treating matters of health and illness is conveyed in a number of texts. See, for example, Briggs, *Manual of Hygiene for Schools and Colleges*; Halpenny and Ireland, *How to be Healthy*, 174; J. Mace Andress and W.A. Evans, *Healthy Citizenship* (Toronto: Ginn and Company, 1935), 63.

27 W.W. Chipman, "The Infant Soldier," *Canadian Nurse* 14 (1918): 1453–63. A number of scholars have focused on experts, mothers, and the state during this period in Canada, Europe, and the United States. Some exemplars of this work include Comacchio, *Nations are Built of Babies*; Katherine Arnup, *Education for Motherhood: Advice for Mothers in Twentieth-Century Canada* (Toronto: University of Toronto Press, 1994); Gisela Bock and Pat Thane, eds., *Maternity and Gender Policies: Women and the Rise of European Welfare States, 1880s to 1950s* (London and New York: Routledge Press, 1994); Molly Ladd-Taylor, *Mother-Work: Women, Child Welfare and the State 1890–1930* (Chicago: University of Illinois Press, 1994).

28 Moore, "Child Welfare Work."

29 Province of British Columbia, *First Report of the Provincial Board of Health* (Victoria: Queen's Printer, 1895), 541–2. Duncan concluded, "Canton, from which the greatest part of Chinese immigration flows to these shores, is regarded as the most filthy city in the world, and is known to be continually impregnated with cholera." 545.

30 "Introductory Report by the Chairman," *Second Report of the Provincial Board of Health* (Victoria: Queen's Printer, 1897), 690.

31 Tim Stanley, "White Supremacy and the Rhetoric of Educational Indoctrination: A Canadian Case Study," in Jean Barman and Mona Gleason, eds., *Children, Teachers, and School in the History of British*

Columbia (Calgary: Detselig Press, 2003), 113–32; and Gleason, "Race, Class, and Health."
32 Sing Lim, *West Coast Chinese Boy* (Montreal: Tundra Books, 1979), 18.
33 Minnie Aodla Freeman, *Life Among the Qallunaat* (Edmonton: Hurtig Publishers, 1978), 98.
34 Donald T. Fraser and George Porter, *Ontario Public School Health Book* (Toronto: Copp Clark Company Ltd., 1925), 11.
35 Neil Sutherland, "The Triumph of 'Formalism': Elementary Schooling in Vancouver from the 1920s to the 1960s," *BC Studies*, (1986) 69–70: 175–210.
36 School nursing grew out of the school medical inspection movement. See Sutherland, *Children in English-Canadian Society*, "Chapter 3: 'Education … Carried on Principally in the Home': The Campaign to Reduce Infant Mortality, 1895–1920"; and Gleason, "Race, Class, and Health."
37 Fraser and Porter, *Ontario Public Health Book*, (preface).
38 Jessie I. Lummis and Williedell Schawe, *The Safety Hill of Health* (New York: World Book Company, 1927), ii.
39 CHP Interview 29, transcript, 7.
40 In the British Columbian context, for example, see Gleason, "Race, Class, and Health." Similarly dire conditions plagued schools in New Zealand at the turn of the century. See Pamela J. Woods, "Hazardous to Children's Health? New Zealand Primary Schools, 1890–1914," *History News* 66 (1993): 4–7.
41 See Gleason, "Race, Class, and Health," 100–1.
42 Ingrid Cowlie, "Memories of the First Wildwood School," in Barbara Ann Lambert, ed., *Chalkdust and Outhouses – Westcoast Schools, 1893–1950* (Powell River: Barbara Lambert, 2000), 110.
43 Kay Hodson, "Malaspina Cranberry Lake School," in Lambert, *Chalkdust and Outhouses*, 118.
44 Robert Collins, *Butter Down the Well – Recollections of a Canadian Childhood* (Saskatoon: Western Producer Prairie Books, 1980), 45.
45 J. Mace Andress, *Wide-Awake School* (Boston: Ginn, 1931), 181.
46 Andress and Breeze, *Health Essentials for Canadian Schools*, 12.
47 CHP Interview 29N, transcript, 8. Emphasis in original interview.
48 CHP Interview 20, transcript 4.
49 T. Wood, M. Lerrigo, and Nina Lamkin, *New Ways for Old* (New York: Newson and Company, 1938).
50 It is also important to note that this curriculum makes equations among healthy bodies, robust citizenship, and able-bodiment. On assumptions regarding able-bodiedness and access to citizenship, see Helen Meekosha

and Leanne Dowse, "Enabling Citizenship: Gender, Disability, and Citizenship in Australia," *Feminist Review* 57 (1997): 49–72.
51 Andress and Breeze, *Health Essentials for Canadian Schools*, 243.
52 Wood et al., *New Ways for Old*, 282.
53 Ibid., 275.
54 Andress, *Wide-Awake School*, 134.
55 Andress and Evans, *Healthy Citizenship*, 51–2.
56 Kelm, *Colonizing Bodies*; Celia Haig-Brown, *Resistance and Renewal: Surviving the Indian Residential School* (Vancouver: Arsenal Pulp Press, 1988); J.R. Miller, *Shingwauk's Vision – A History of Native Residential Schools* (Toronto: University of Toronto Press, 1996); J.S. Milloy, *National Crime: Canadian Government and the Residential School System, 1879 to 1976* (Winnipeg: University of Manitoba Press, 1999).
57 Freeman, *Life Among the Qallunaat*, 104.
58 Kelm, *Colonizing Bodies*, see especially "Chapter 4: A 'Scandalous Procession': Residential Schooling and the Reformation of Aboriginal Bodies," 57–80.
59 On the racialization of Canadian citizenship, see Claude Denis, "Indigenous Citizenship and History in Canada: Between Denial and Imposition," in Robert Adamoski, Dorothy E. Chunn, and Robert Menzies, eds., *Contesting Canadian Citizenship – Historical Readings* (Peterborough: Broadview Press, 2002), 113–26.
60 Freeman, *Life Among the Qallunaat*, 125.
61 Marion Gallagher, "School Days in Victoria," in Lambert, *Chalkdust and Outhouses*, 276.
62 Collins, *Butter Down the Well*, 42.
63 CHP Interview 03N, transcript, 9.
64 CHP Interview 02N, transcript, 1.
65 CHP Interview 22, transcript, 17.

CHAPTER FIVE

1 The Hospital for Sick Children (HSC), nicknamed Sick Kids, was founded in 1875 and was the "first hospital in Canada designed specifically for the care of sick children." Judith Young, "'Little Sufferers': Sick Children in Late-Nineteenth Century Toronto," *Nursing History Review* 3 (1995): 129.
2 All patient names have been changed.
3 Alan Brown, "The Ability of Mothers to Nurse Their Infants," *Canadian Medical Association Journal* 7, 3 (March, 1917): 241–7; Alan Brown,

"Problems of the Rural Mother in the Feeding of her Children," *Public Health Journal* 9, 7 (July, 1918): 297–301; Alan Brown, *The Normal Child – Its Care and Feeding* (New York: Century Company, 1923). On Alan Brown's contributions to the invention of Pablum, for which Toronto's HSC still receives royalties, see *http://www.sickkids.ca/abouthsc/custom/brown.asp* (Retrieved 12 December 2007)

4 *http://www.mta.ca/about_canada/study_guide/doctors/better_foods.html* (Retrieved 27 May 2008).

5 HSC Patient Records, Microfiche Index 1001–1655, box 1, 1914–1916. Records no. 1014, 1053, 1016, 3334, 3335, 3628, 3031, 1011.

6 Young, "'Young Sufferers'"; Heather Munro Prescott, *A Doctor of Their Own: A History of Adolescent Medicine* (Cambridge, MA: Harvard University Press, 1998). Stang and Joshi, "The Evolution of Freestanding Children's Hospitals in Canada."

7 On the development of publicly funded health services in Canada in the post-Second World War era, see Naylor, *Private Practice, Public Payment.*

8 See for example Young, "'Young Sufferers'"; Paul Gagan, *A Necessity Among Us: The Owen Sound General and Marine Hospital, 1981–1985* (Toronto: University of Toronto Press, 1990); Paul Gagan and Rosemary Gagan, *For Patients of Moderate Means: A Social History of the Voluntary Public General Hospital in Canada, 1890 to 1950* (Montreal & Kingston: McGill-Queen's University Press, 2002); Heather MacDougall, *Activists and Advocates: Toronto's Health Department, 1883–1983* (Toronto: Dundurn Press, 1990). In the United States, Heather Munro Prescott's groundbreaking history of the development of adolescent medicine usefully includes the perspectives of patients, gathered primarily through letters from teenagers and parents, particularly in chapter 3. Prescott, *A Doctor of Their Own.*

9 Baillargeon, "Learning and Leisure on the Inside" in Gleason et al., *Lost Kids*, 117–35.

10 Annmarie Adams, *Medicine by Design: The Architect and the Modern Hospital, 1893–1943* (Minneapolis: University of Minnesota Press, 2008). See "Chapter 2: Patients."

11 Partington's analysis is based on the admission of 2,226 children aged fourteen and under (out of a total 12,759) between 1 October 1899 and 30 September 1909. M.W. Partington, "Paediatric Admissions to Kingston General Hospital, Kingston, Ontario (1889–1909)," *Families* 22, 1 (1983): 33–46.

12 On contagious disease prevention efforts, see chapter 1.

13 M.W. Partington, "Paediatric Admissions to Kingston General Hospital," 33–46.

14 Florence C. Moffatt, "Forgotten Villages of the BC Coast – Hospital Life at Bella Bella," *Raincoast Chronicles* 11 (1987): 52.
15 Comacchio, *Nations Are Built of Babies*; Wendy Mitchinson, *Giving Birth in Canada, 1900–1950* (Toronto: University of Toronto Press, 2002).
16 Comacchio, *Nations Are Built of Babies*, 21–5.
17 On the development of more formalized ties between public health advocates and hospital in the early decades of the twentieth century, see Heather MacDougall, *Activists and Advocates: Toronto's Health Department, 1883–1983* (Dundurn Press: Toronto, 1990). On Brown's research at the HSC see L. Bruce Robertson and Alan Brown, "Blood Transfusion in Infants and Young Children," *Canadian Medical Association Journal* 54 (April, 1915): 298–305; Alan Brown, "Duodenal Ulcers in Infancy," *Canadian Medical Association Journal* 74 (April, 1917): 320–3; Alan Brown, George E. Smith, and Gordon Phillips, "Auto-Serum Treatment of Chorea," *Canadian Medical Association Journal* 91 (January, 1919): 52–62; Alan Brown, "Some Factors Concerning the Care of the Newborn," *Canadian Public Health Journal* 29, 7 (July, 1938): 337–44; Nelles Silverthorne, Alan Brown, and W. J. Auger, "Pneumonia in Childhood," *Canadian Medical Association Journal* 44, 5 (May, 1941): 492–6; Alan Brown and Elizabeth Chant Richardson, "Essential Features Concerning the Proper Nutrition of the Infant and Child," *Canadian Medical Association Journal* 48, 4 (April, 1943): 297–302; John R. Ross and Alan Brown, "Poisonings Common in Children," *Canadian Medical Association Journal* 64, 4 (April 1951): 285–8.
18 Baillargeon, "Learning and Leisure on the Inside."
19 Judith Young, "Changing Attitudes Towards Families of Hospitalized Children from 1935 to 1975: A Case Study," *Journal of Advanced Nursing* 17 (1992): 1422–9. Young points out that "regulations were considerably less restrictive for the small number of private patients."
20 Ibid.
21 W.W. Bauer, "Childhood's #1 Enemy," *Maclean's* magazine 14 September 1946, 46. On the post-Second World War popularity of psychology as an explanatory discourse for behaviour of young people in Canada see Mona Gleason, *Normalizing the Ideal: Psychology, Schooling and the Family in Postwar Canada* (Toronto: University of Toronto Press, 1999); Mary Louise Adams, *The Trouble With Normal – Postwar Youth and the Making of Heterosexuality* (Toronto: University of Toronto Press, 1997).
22 Alice Buckhardt, "Play While you Nurse," *The Canadian Nurse* 33, 2 (December, 1937): 591.
23 Ibid., 593.
24 Ibid.

25 Esme M. Baker, "Enuresis," *The Canadian Nurse* 51, 9 (September, 1955), 712.
26 Child Health Project (CHP), Interview 008N, transcript, 5.
27 Françoise Miller Ouellet, "Play Therapy and the Nurse," *The Canadian Nurse* 56, 4 (April 1960): 346.
28 Like the oral history participants, all names from HSC patient records have been changed.
29 HSC Patient Records, record 59060, 2 October 1930.
30 CHP, Interview 11N, transcript, 3. All names are pseudonyms.
31 CHP, Interview 29N, transcript, 3.
32 CHP, Interview 021N, transcript, 4–5.
33 CHP, Interview 2, transcript, 5.
34 CHP, Interview 6, transcript, 8.
35 CHP, Interview 19, transcript, 12.
36 CHP, Interview 011, transcript, 10.
37 Ibid., 11.
38 CHP, Interview 6, transcript 2.
39 Ibid., 7.
40 CHP, Interview 03N, transcript, 6.

CHAPTER SIX

1 Ellen Key, *The Century of the Child* (New York: J.P. Putnam's Sons, 1909). Portions of this chapter were first published in Gleason, "Navigating the Pedagogy of Failure: Medicine, Education and the Disabled Child in English Canada, 1900–1945," in Nathanael Lauster and Graham Allan, eds., *The End of Children? Changing Trends in Childbearing and Childhood* (Vancouver: UBC Press, 2012), 140–60.
2 Andrew Jones and Leonard Rutman, *In the Children's Aid: J.J. Kelso and Child Welfare in Ontario* (Toronto: University of Toronto Press, 1981); Sutherland, *Children in English-Canadian Society*; Myers, *Caught*; Tamara Myers and Joan Sangster, "Retorts, Runaways, and Riots: Patterns of Resistance in Canadian Reform Schools for Girls, 1930–1960," *Journal of Social History* 34:3 (Spring 2001): 669–98.
3 Three important conceptual and interpretive points are at play in this chapter: 1) Although considered derisive to modern ears, the terms I use such as "defective," "degeneracy," "crippled," and "feeble-minded" are those used by the professional in the past and require careful historical unpacking. 2) Not all children labeled disabled in the past would be labeled thus contemporarily, and vice versa. 3) By employing quotation marks around

particular words and phrases, for example, "defective" and "handicap,' it is my intention to trouble them, suggest their social construction, and open them up to historical inquiry.

4 I surveyed leading professional medical journals for doctors and nurses, including the *Canadian Medical Association Journal*, and the *Public Health Journal* over the first four decades of the twentieth century. I also used health textbooks that were approved for use in English Canadian schools over the period.

5 *http://easterseals.ca/english/* (Retrieved 10 February 2012)

6 Paul Longmore, "The Cultural Framing of Disability: The Telethon as a Case Study," *PMLA* 120, 2 (March 2005): 502–8; Rosemarie Garland, "Seeing the Disabled: Visual Rhetorics of Disability in Popular Photography," in Paul Longmore and Lauri Umansky, eds., *The New Disability History: American Perspectives* (New York: New York University Press, 2001), 335–74.

7 Michael T. Hayes and Rhonda S. Black, "Troubling Signs: Disability, Hollywood Movies and the Construction of a Discourse of Pity," *Disability Studies Quarterly* 22, 3 (2003): 114–32.

8 Scholars such as Gerald Thomson, Nic Clarke, Jessa Chupik, David Wright, and Veronica Strong-Boag have focused on judgements of various educational, medical, and social work professionals regarding disability. Gerald Thomson, "A Fondness for Charts and Children: Scientific Progressivism in Vancouver Schools 1920 to 1950," *Historical Studies in Education*, 12, 1/2 (2002): 111–28; Gerald Thomson, "'Through No Fault of Their Own': Josephine Dauphinee and the 'Subnormal' Pupils of the Vancouver School System, 1911–1941," *Historical Studies in Education* 18, 1 (2006): 51–73; Nic Clarke, "Sacred Daemons: Exploring British Columbian Society's Perceptions of 'Mentally Deficient' Children, 1870–1930," *BC Studies* 144 (Winter 04/05): 61–90; Jessa Chupik, "Fires Burning: Advocacy, Camping and Children with Learning Disabilities in Ontario, 1950–1990," in Duncan Mitchell, Rannveig Trautadottir, Rohhss Chapman, Louise Townson, Nigel Ingham, and Sue Ledger, eds., *Exploring Experiences of Advocacy by People with Learning Disabilities* (London: Jessica Kingsley Publishers, 2006): 119–27; Jessa Chupik and David Wright, "Treating the 'Idiot' Child in Early Twentieth-Century Ontario," *Disability & Society* 21, 1 (January 2006): 77–90; Veronica Strong-Boag, "'Today's Child': Preparing for the 'Just Society' One Family at a Time,' Canadian Historical Review 86, 4 (December 2005): 673–99.

9 Michel Foucault, "The subject and power," in H.L. Dreyfus and P. Rabinow, eds., *Michel Foucault: Beyond Structuralism and Hermeneutics* (Brighton, Sussex: The Harvester Press, 1986), 208–26.

10 Nic Clarke, "Sacred Daemons: Exploring British Columbian Society's Perceptions of 'Mentally Deficient' Children, 1870–1930," *BC Studies* 144 (Winter 04/05): 64.
11 Ibid.
12 I use four oral history interviews in this chapter. On the role of oral history in this book, see the introduction for details of the oral history project and associated limits of using oral history testimony in historical accounts.
13 David Mitchell and Sharon Snyder have encouraged historians to pay more interpretive attention to the role of eugenic science – the belief that limiting the "breeding of undesirables" helped ameliorate social problems – in expressions of mass violence, genocide, and marginalization of "otherness" from the late eighteenth century to at least the end of the Second World War. See David Mitchell and Sharon Snyder, "The Eugenic Atlantic: race, disability, and the making of an international Eugenic science, 1800–1945," *Disability & Society* 18, 7 (December 2003): 843–64.
14 Harvey G. Simmons, *From Asylum to Welfare* (Toronto: National Institute on Mental Retardation, 1982), Angus MacLaren, *Our Own Master Race – Eugenics in Canada, 1885–1945* (Toronto: Oxford University Press, 1990); Nic Clarke, "Sacred Daemons," 61–90; James W. Trent, *Inventing the Feeble Mind: A History of Mental Retardation in the United States* (Berkeley: University of California Press, 1994); Daniel J. Kevles, *In the Name of Eugenics: Genetics and the Uses of Human Heredity* (New York: Knopf, 1985); Martin S. Pernick, *The Black Stork: Eugenics and the Death of "Defective" Babies in American Medicine and the Motion Pictures Since 1915* (New York: Oxford University Press, 1996); Mark Adams, ed., *The Wellborn Science: Eugenics in Germany, France, Brazil and Russia* (New York: Oxford University Press, 1990); Christopher Kliewer and Linda May Fitzgerald, "Disability, Schooling and the Artifacts of Colonialism," *Teachers College Record* 103, 3 (June 2001): 450–70.
15 See MacLaren, "Chapter 1: The Birth of Biological Politics," in *Our Own Master*, 13–27 for a detailed accounting of the broad and powerful coalition of social reformers who advocated eugenics thinking at the turn of the twentieth century.
16 C.K. Clarke, "The Evolution of Imbecility," *Queen's Quarterly* 6, 4 (April 1899): 297–314. Charles K. Clarke was the father of Eric Kirk Clarke.
17 Ibid., 306.
18 G.S. Mundie, "The Mentally Defective," *Canadian Medical Association Journal* 4, 5 (May, 1914): 398.
19 Anonymous, "Defective Children Product of Neglect," *Victoria Daily Times*, 14 May 1920, 6.

20 See MacLaren, *Our Own Master Race*.
21 As Deborah Park and John Radford have shown, judgments of the hospitals' eugenics boards and allied professionals guided individual decisions to sterilize. D. Park and J. Radforth, "From the Case Files: Reconstructing a History of Forced Sterilization," *Disability and Society* 13, 3 (June 1998): 317–42.
22 MacLaren, *Our Own Master Race*, 146–48.
23 Chupik and Wright, "Treating the 'Idiot' Child in Early Twentieth-Century Ontario."
24 Hector Charles Cameron, "Sleep and its Disorders in Childhood," *Canadian Medical Association Journal* 24, 2 (February 1931): 240.
25 Lloyd P. MacHaffie, "Preventative Pediatrics as seen by the School Medical Officer," *Canadian Public Health Journal* 28, 10 (October 1937): 498.
26 Harold Sutherland, "Health of the Baby Becomes Increasingly Important," *Saturday Night* (23 March 1940): 17.
27 Ibid., 17.
28 Ibid., 22.
29 Harris McPhedran, "The Pre-School Child," *Canadian Medical Association Journal* 20, 6 (June 1929): 659.
30 HSC, Patient Record, record 29349, 4 April 1922.
31 CHP, Interview 017, transcript, 6–7.
32 D.J. Dunn, "Medical Inspection of School Children," *Canadian Medical Association Journal* 8, 10 (October, 1918): 932.
33 See Jason Ellis, "'Backward and Brilliant Children': A Social and Policy History of Disability, Childhood, and Education in Toronto's Special Education Classes, 1910 to 1945," PhD thesis, OISE, University of Toronto, 2011; Angus MacLaren, *Our Own Master Race*; Gerald Thomson, "A Fondness for Charts and Children"; Gerald Thomson, "'Through No Fault of Their Own': Josephine Dauphinee and the 'Subnormal' Pupils of the Vancouver School System, 1911–1941"; Clarke, "Sacred Daemons." The influence of eugenic reasoning in justifications for the institutionalization and sterilizing of the "feeble-minded" found multinational expressions. See, for example, James W. Trent, *Inventing the feeble mind: A history of mental retardation in the United States* (Berkeley: University of California Press, 1994), and Christopher Kliewer and Linda May Fitzgerald, "Disability, Schooling and the Artifacts of Colonialism," *Teachers College Record* 103, 3 (June 2001): 450–70.
34 On Dauphinee's contribution to the institutionalization imperative surrounding children labeled mentally "defective," see Thomson's "Through No Fault of Their Own."

35 A.P. Knight, *The Ontario Public School Hygiene* (Toronto: Copp Clark Limited, 1910), 229.
36 Mundie, "The Mentally Defective," 399.
37 Ibid., 404.
38 D.J. Dunn, "Medical Inspection of School Children," 928.
39 See Ellis, "Backward and Brilliant Children," (introduction). See also F. Armstrong, "The Historical Development of Special Education: Humanitarian Rationality or 'Wild Profusion of Entangled Events'? *History of Education* 31, 5 (2002): 437–56; J. Read and J. Walmsley, "Historical perspectives on special education, 1890–1970," *Disability & Society* 21, 5 (2006): 455–69.
40 Thomson, "Through No Fault of Their Own," 55–6. See also Trent, *Inventing the Feeble Mind*.
41 MacMurchy, "The Mentally Defective Child," 86.
42 G. S. Mundie, "Juvenile Delinquency," *Canadian Medical Association Journal* 5, 5 (May 1915): 405.
43 MacMurchy, "The Mentally Defective Child," *Public Health Journal* 6, 2 (February, 1915): 86.
44 Mrs. M.H. Kerr, "Defective Children," *Public Health Journal* 6, 12 (December 1915): 620.
45 In the interwar period, equations between what was judged "failures of development" with racial inferiority were perhaps most explicitly exemplified by professional characteristics of "Mongolism" or Down's syndrome. Hegemonic ideas about race dictated that the "races of mankind" were arranged hierarchically with "Caucasians" at the top and "Mongolians" at the bottom. Other groups, such as the "Ethiopian," "Malaysian," and "American (American continent)," occupied middle positions. Human embryos, scientific thinking held, retraced or recapitulated the phases of the evolutionary history of its race as it developed in the womb. Thus, Langdon Down, the British doctor who provided the first comprehensive description of this "deficiency," labelled the physical features associated with the syndrome as representing "Mongol" – lower race – features. See, for example, the discussion in Elizabeth M. Warner, "A Survey of Mongolism, with a Review of One Hundred Cases," *Canadian Medical* Association *Journal* 33, 5 (November 1935): 495–500. Useful historical critiques are offered in Peter Volpe, "Is Down Syndrome a Modern Disease?" *Perspectives in Biology and Medicine* 29, 3 Part 1 (Spring 1986): 423–36; Stephen J. Gould, "Dr. Down's Syndrome," *Natural History* 89, 4 (1980): 142–8.
46 For more details on Florence, see chapter 2.
47 CHP, Interview 023, transcript, 1–5.
48 For more details on Theresa, see chapter 2.

49 CHP, Interview 10, transcript, 4.
50 CHP, Interview 24, transcript, 9.
51 Robin Williams, *A Vancouver Boyhood – Reflections of Growing up in Vancouver, 1925–1945* (Vancouver: Peanut Butter Publishing, 1997), 199.
52 Patricia Vertinsky, "The Social Construction of the Gendered Body: Exercise and the Exercise of Power," *International Journal of the History of Sport* 11 (August 1994): 147–71.
53 J. Mace Andress, I. Goldberger, Marguerite P. Dolch, *Growing Big and Strong* (Boston: Ginn and Company, 1939), 49.
54 CHP, Interview 10, transcript, 8.
55 J. Mace Andress and Elizabeth Breeze, *Health Essentials for High School*, 242.
56 Ibid., 6
57 Andress et al., *Growing Big and Strong*, 121.
58 Geoffrey Hayes, "Science and the Magic Eye: Innovations in the Selection of Canadian Army Officers, 1939–1945," *Armed Forces and Society* 22, 2 (Winter 1995): 275–95.
59 See chapter 5 in this book.
60 Hamilton Baxter, "Plastic Correction of Protruding Ears in Children," *Canadian Medical Association Journal* (September 1941): 217–20.
61 Ibid., 217.
62 Ross A. Campbell, "The Spastic Child," *Canadian Nurse* 42, 6 (June, 1946): 469–73.
63 Donald Paterson, "Health Services for Handicapped Child in British Columbia," *Canadian Medical Association Journal* 76, 6 (15 March 1957): 483–85.
64 CHP, Interview 015, transcript, 7.

CONCLUSION

1 HSC, Patient Records, record 87519, 23 August 1937.
2 Veronica Strong-Boag, "'Children of Adversity': Disability and Child Welfare in Canada from the Nineteenth to the Twenty-First Century," *Journal of Family History* 32, 4 (2007): 424.
3 Veronica Strong-Boag, *Fostering Nation? Canada Confronts Its History of Childhood Disadvantage* (Waterloo: Wilfrid University Press, 2010).
4 Wendy Mitchinson, *The Nature of their Bodies: Women and Their Doctors in Victorian Canada* (Toronto: University of Toronto Press, 1991).
5 See Mary-Ellen Kelm, *Colonizing Bodies: Aboriginal Health and Healing in British Columbia, 1900–1950* (Vancouver: UBC Press, 1999).

6 Claudia Castaneda, *Figuration: Child, Bodies, Worlds* (Durham and London: Duke University Press, 2002), 1. Social scientists in a variety of disciplines, most particularly sociology and anthropology, have been increasingly critical of this "developmental" conception of children, discounting as it does the social and historical contexts in which children grow up. Called the "new social studies of childhood," this massive body of literature challenges the conceptualization of children as primarily bound by developmental and biologically based changes. The field has, in recent years, also itself been criticized for perpetuating its own binary approaches to childhood. In this case, the "social" has come to function in much the same way as the "biological." See Alan Prout, *The Future of Childhood – Towards the Interdisciplinary Study of Children* (London and New York: Routledge Farmer, 2005). In terms of its relationship to history, see Patrick Ryan, "How 'New' is the New Sociology of Childhood: The Myth of a Paradigm Shift," *Journal of Interdisciplinary History* 38, 4 (Spring 2008): 553–76.

7 CHP, Interview 013, transcript, 1.

8 Ibid., transcript, 7.

9 Robert MacIntosh, "Constructing the Child: New Approaches to the History of Childhood in Canada," *Acadiensis* 18, 2 (Spring 1999): 128.

10 See, for example, the Government of Canada, *Report of the Royal Commission on Aboriginal People* (1996).

11 See, for example, Canadian Institute of Child Health, *The Health of Canada's Children: A CICH Profile* (Ottawa: Canadian Institute of Child Health, 1989); Canadian Institute of Child Health, *The Health of Canada's Children: A CICH Profile, 2nd Edition* (Ottawa: Canadian Institute of Child Health, 1994); Canadian Institute of Child Health, *The Health of Canada's Children: A CICH Profile, 3rd Edition* (Ottawa: Canadian Institute of Child Health, 2000); Elizabeth Shaw and Danielle Grenier, "Taking the pulse of Canadian children – a health report card for the millennium," *Paediatric Children Health* 6, 4 (April 2001): 181–3. On the neglect of disadvantaged children, see Gleason et al., "Introduction," *Lost Kids*.

12 Standing Senate Committee on Social Affairs, Science and Technology, Report of the Subcommittee on Cities, *In from the Margins: A Call to Action on Poverty, Housing and Homelessness* (2009), 6–7.

13 Kim Pemberton, "Health officer cites shocking statistics on B.C. child poverty," *Vancouver Sun* 17 June 1998, A1–A2.

14 First Call: BC Child and Youth Advocacy Coalition, "BC Campaign 2000 – 2010 Child Poverty Report Card." *www.firstcallbc.org* (Retrieved 17 May 2011)

Selected Bibliography

ARCHIVAL SOURCES

Hospital for Sick Children (HSC) Patient Records, Microfiche Index 1001–1655, box 1, 1914–1916. Records no. 1014, 1053, 1016, 3334, 3335, 3628, 3031, 1011.

Library and Archives Canada (LAC), MG 28 I 343, Canadian Medical Association (CMA), Volume 7, File 1, Minutes (book) CMA Section of Public Health, "Report of the Pediatric Section of the CMA, June 18, 1924," 73.

ORAL HISTORY INTERVIEWS

Bonner, Katherine. 2005. CHP Interview 017. 12 May.
Brand, Shirley. 2005. CHP Interview 1. 14 January.
Brennan, John. 2005. CHP Interview 14. 2 May.
Cameron, Mark. 2004. CHP Interview 20. 25 August.
Clarke, Mattie. 2005 CHP Interview 04N. 27 April.
Colussi, Lina. 2005. CHP Interview 32. 6 September.
Davies, Eileen. 2004. CHP Interview 03N. 27 February.
Dearland, Janie. 2004. CHP Interview 18N. 25 August.
Desjardin, Amelia. 2005. CHP Interview 013. 25 April.
Drake, Florence. 2005. CHP Interview 023. 9 July.
Elliott, Theresa. 2005. CHP Interview 10. 30 April.
Friedman, Irena. 2003. CHP Interview 2. 26 January.
Itou, Megumi. 2006. CHP Interview 40. 26 May.
Johnson, Frank. 2004. CHP Interview 02N. 26 February.
Knott, Andrea. 2004. CHP Interview 11N. 28 July.
Lockhart, Agnes. 2005. CHP Interview 24. 10 July.

Lossky, Bill. 2005. CHP Interview 015. 2 May.
MacKenzie, Doris. 2005. CHP Interview 22. 7 June.
Mason, Lily. 2005. CHP Interview 4. 10 February.
Mercer, Alice. 2004. CHP Interview 5. 7 April.
Moss, Kyle. 2004. CHP Interview 007N. 29 April.
Myers, Glenda. 2004. CHP Interview 10N. 28 July.
McCrea, Jack. 2005. CHP Interview 7A. 23 February.
Price, Trisha. 2005. CHP Interview 19. 15 May.
Randall, Jenny. 2004. CHP Interview 29N. 29 September.
Rupert, Gladys. 2005. CHP Interview 011. 11 March.
Sweeney, William. 2005. CHP Interview 008N. 10 June.
Sutherland, Kathryn. 2004. CHP Interview 06N. 15 April.
Tilley, Catherine. 2005. CHP Interview 8. 4 March.
Trapier, Marc. 2004. CHP Interview 024. 26 August.
Traster, Donald. 2005. CHP Interview 6. 10 February.
Welsh, Monica. 2004. CHP Interview 021N. 26 August.

PRINTED SOURCES

Adamoski, Robert, Dorothy E. Chunn, and Robert Menzies, eds. *Contesting Canadian Citizenship – Historical Readings*. Peterborough: Broadview Press, 2002.
Adams, Annmarie. *Medicine by Design: The Architect and the Modern Hospital, 1893–1943*. Minneapolis: University of Minnesota Press, 2008.
– and David Theodore. "Children's Hospitals in Toronto and Montreal, 1875–2006." *Canadian Bulletin of Medical History* 19, 1 (2002): 201–43.
Adams, Mark, ed. *The Wellborn Science: Eugenics in Germany, France, Brazil and Russia*. New York: Oxford University Press, 1990.
Adams, Mary Louise. *The Trouble with Normal – Postwar Youth and the Making of Heterosexuality*. Toronto: University of Toronto Press, 1997.
Altenbaugh, Richard J. "Where are the Disabled in the History of Education? The Impact of Polio on Sites of Learning." *History of Education* 35, 6 (November 2006): 705–30.
Andress, J. Mace, I. Goldberger, and Marguerite Dolch. *Growing Big and Strong – Safe and Healthy Living Series*. Boston: Ginn and Company, 1939.
Anonymous. "The Health of the Child." *Canadian Medical Association Journal* 2, 8 (August 1912): 704–5.
Anonymous. "Health Centre Work a Living Memorial." *Victoria Daily Times* (21 August 1919): 18.
Anonymous. "Defective Children Product of Neglect." *Victoria Daily Times* (14 May 1920): 6.

Ansley, H.A. "State of Health of People of Canada, 1945." *Canadian Journal of Public Health* 38, 6 (June 1947): 271–3.
Apple, Michael W., and Linda K. Christian-Smith, eds. *The Politics of the, Textbook*. New York: Routledge, 1991.
Armstrong, David. "The Invention of Infant Mortality." *Sociology of Health and Illness* 8 (1986): 211–32.
Armstrong, F. "The Historical Development of Special Education: Humanitarian Rationality or 'Wild Profusion of Entangled Events'?" *History of Education* 31, 5 (2002): 437–56.
Arnup, Katherine. 1992. "Victims of Vaccination?": Opposition to Compulsory Immunization in Ontario, 1900–90." *Canadian Bulletin of Medical History* 9: 159–76.
Ashby, Henry, and G.A. Wright. *The Diseases of Children – Medical and Surgical*. New York: Longmans, Green and Company Medical Publishers, 1897.
Baillargeon, Denyse. *Babies for the Nation: The Medicalization of Motherhood in Quebec, 1910–1970*. Translated by W. Donald Wilson. Waterloo: Wilfrid Laurier University Press, 2009.
Baker, Esme M. "Enuresis." *The Canadian Nurse* 51, 9 (September, 1955): 712–14.
Baldus, Bernd, and Meenaz Kassam. "'Make me truthful, good and mild': Values in Nineteenth-century Ontario Schoolbooks." *Canadian Journal of Sociology* 21 (1996): 327–58.
Bareto, Luis, and Christopher Rutty. "The Speckled Monster: Canada, Small pox, and its Eradication." *Canadian Journal of Public Health* 93, 4 (2002): 12–30.
Barman, Jean, and Mona Gleason, eds. *Children, Teachers, and School in the History of British Columbia*. Calgary: Detselig Press, 2003.
Bauer, W.W. "Childhood's #1 Enemy." *Maclean's* magazine (14 September 1946): 46–7.
Baxter, Hamilton. "Plastic Correction of Protruding Ears in Children." *Canadian Medical Association Journal* (September 1941): 217–20.
Bell, Robert. *The "Medicine-Man," or, Indian and Eskimo Notions of Medicine*. Montreal: Gazette Printing Company, 1886.
Bock, Gisela, and Pat Thane, eds. *Maternity and Gender Policies: Women and the Rise of European Welfare States, 1880s to 1950s*. London and New York: Routledge Press, 1994.
Bourgeois, Charles E. *The Protection of Children in the Province of Quebec*. Translated by Paul E. Marquis. Trois-Rivieres: M. Roy, 1948.
Boyd, Helen. "Growing Up Privileged in Edmonton." *Alberta History* 30, 1 (1982): 1–10.

Briggs, William. *Manual of Hygiene for Schools and Colleges*. Toronto: Provincial Board of Health, 1886.
British Columbia Department of Health. "Introductory Report by the Chairman." *Second Report of the Provincial Board of Health*, 689–99. Victoria: Queen's Printer, 1897.
Brown, Alan. "The Ability of Mothers to Nurse Their Infants." *Canadian Medical Association Journal* 7, 3 (March 1917): 241–7.
– "Duodenal Ulcers in Infancy." *Canadian Medical Association Journal* 74 (April 1917): 320–3.
– "Problems of the Rural Mother in the Feeding of her Children." *Public Health Journal* 9, 7 (July 1918): 297–301.
– George E. Smith, and Gordon Phillips. "Auto-Serum Treatment of Chorea." *Canadian Medical Association Journal* 91 (January 1919): 52–62.
– *The Normal Child – Its Care and Feeding*. New York: Century Company, 1923.
– "Some Factors Concerning the Care of the Newborn." *Canadian Public Health Journal* 29, 7 (July 1938): 337–44.
– and Elizabeth Chant Richardson. "Essential Features Concerning the Proper Nutrition of the Infant and Child." *Canadian Medical Association Journal* 48, 4 (April 1943): 297–302.
Browne, Jean. "School Nursing in Regina." *Canadian Nurse* 7, 9 (September 1911): 439–45.
Brownlie, Robin Jarvis. "'Living the Same as White People': Mohawk and Anishinabe Women's Labour in Southern Ontario, 1920–1940." *Labour/Le Travail* 61 (Spring 2008): 41–68.
Buckhardt, Alice. "Play While you Nurse." *The Canadian Nurse* 33, 2 (December 1937): 590–3.
Cameron, Agnes Deans. "Parent and Teacher." *Canadian Magazine of Politics, Science, Art and Literature* XV (May-October 1900): 538.
Campbell, Hector Charles. *Diseases of Childhood – A Short Introduction*. London: Oxford University Press, 1926.
Campbell, Ross A. "The Spastic Child." *Canadian Nurse* 42 (1946): 471–4.
Canadian Institute of Child Health. *The Health of Canada's Children: A CICH Profile*. Ottawa: Canadian Institute of Child Health, 1989.
– *The Health of Canada's Children: A CICH Profile, 2nd Edition*. Ottawa: Canadian Institute of Child Health, 1994.
– *The Health of Canada's Children: A CICH Profile, 3rd Edition*. Ottawa: Canadian Institute of Child Health, 2000.

Carstairs, Catherine, and Rachel Elder. "Expertise, Health, and Popular Opinion: Debating Water Fluoridation, 1945–1980." *Canadian Historical Review* 89, 3 (September 2008): 345–71.

Chavasse, Pye Henry. *Advice to a Mother on the Management of Her Children and on the Treatment on the Moment of Some of Their More Pressing Illnesses and Accidents*. Toronto: Willing and Williamson, 1880.

Chipman, W.W. "The Infant Soldier." *Canadian Nurse* 14 (1918): 1453–63.

Christie, Nancy. *Households of Faith – Family, Gender, and Community in Canada, 1760–1969*. Kingston and Montreal: McGill-Queen's University Press, 2002.

– *Engendering the State: Family, Work, and Welfare in Canada*. Toronto: University of Toronto Press, 2000.

Chudacoff, Howard P. *How Old are You? Age Consciousness in American Culture*. New Jersey: Princeton University Press, 1989.

Chupik, Jessa, and David Wright. "Treating the 'Idiot' Child in Early Twentieth-Century Ontario." *Disability & Society* 21, 1 (January 2006): 77–90.

Clarke, C.K. "The Evolution of Imbecility." *Queen's Quarterly* 6, 4 (April 1899): 297–314.

Clarke, Nic. "Sacred Daemons: Exploring British Columbian Society's Perceptions of 'Mentally Deficient' Children, 1870–1930." *BC Studies* 144 (Winter 2004–05): 61–90.

Coe, Richard. *When the Grass was Taller – Autobiography and the Experience of Childhood*. New Haven: Yale University Press, 1984.

Cohn, Victor. *Sister Kenny: The Woman Who Challenged the Doctors*. Burns and MacEachern Limited: Don Mills, 1975.

Collins, Robert. *Butter Down the Well – Recollections of a Canadian Childhood*. Saskatoon: Western Producer Prairie Books, 1980.

Collins-Williams, C. "Accidents in Children." *Canadian Medical Association Journal* 65, 6 (December 1951): 534.

Colón, A.R., with P.A. Colón. *Nurturing Children – A History of Pediatrics*. Westport, CT: Greenwood Press, 1999.

Comacchio, Cynthia R. *Nations are Built of Babies: Saving Ontario's Mothers and Children, 1900–1940*. Montreal and Kingston: McGill-Queen's University Press, 1993.

Couture, Ernest. "Some Aspects of the Child Health Program in Canada." *Canadian Public Health Journal* 30, 12 (December 1939): 580–4.

Crawford, P.R. "Fifty Years of Fluoridation." *Journal – Canadian Dental Association* 61, 7 (1995): 585–8.

Davis, Angela. "'Oh, no, nothing, we didn't learn anything': Sex Education and the Preparation of Girls for Motherhood, c. 1930–1970." *History of Education* 37, 5 (September 2008): 661–77.

Dewhirst, John. "Coast Salish Summer Festivals: Rituals for Upgrading Social Identity." *Anthropologica* 17, 2 (1976): 231–73.

Dreyfus, H.L., and P. Rabinow, eds. *Michel Foucault: Beyond Structuralism and Hermeneutics*. Brighton, Sussex: The Harvester Press, 1986.

Duffy, Jacalyn. *History of Medicine – A Scandalously Short Introduction*. Toronto: University of Toronto Press, 1999.

Dunn, D.J. "Medical Inspection of School Children." *Canadian Medical Association Journal* 8, 10 (October 1918): 926, 932.

Ferland, Jacques. "In Search of the Unbound Prometheia: A Comparative View of Women's Activism in Two Quebec Industries, 1869–1908." *Labour/Le Travail* 24 (Spring 1989): 11–44.

Feudtner, John Christopher. *Bittersweet: Diabetes, Insulin, and the Transformation of Illness*. Chapel Hill: University of North Carolina Press, 2003.

Fife, Austin E. "Popular Legends of the Mormons." *California Folklore Quarterly* 1, 2 (April 1942): 105–25.

First Call: BC Child and Youth Advocacy Coalition. "BC Campaign 2000–2010 Child Poverty Report Card," 2011. *www.firstcallbc.org* (Retrieved 17 May 2011).

Fleming, A. Grant. "The Value of Periodic Health Examinations." *The Canadian Nurse* 25, 6 (June 1929).

Fraser, Donald T. and George Porter. *Ontario Public School Health Book*. Toronto: Copp Clark Company Ltd, 1925.

Freeman, Minnie Aodla. *Life Among the Qallunaat*. Edmonton: Hurtig Publishers, 1978.

Foucault, Michel. "The Subject and Power." *Critical Inquiry* 8, 4 (Summer 1982): 777–95.

Gagan, Paul. *A Necessity Among Us: The Owen Sound General and Marine Hospital, 1981–1985*. Toronto: University of Toronto Press, 1990.

– and Rosemary Gagan. *For Patients of Moderate Means: A Social History of the Voluntary Public General Hospital in Canada, 1890 to 1950*. Montreal and Kingston: McGill-Queen's University Press, 2002.

Gage, W.J. *Gage's Health Series for Intermediate Classes* Part 2. Toronto: W.J. Gage & Company's Educational Series, 1896.

Gleason, Mona. "Embodied Negotiations: Children's Bodies and Historical Change in Canada, 1930–1960." *Journal of Canadian Studies* 34, 1 (Spring 1999): 113–37.

- *Normalizing the Ideal: Psychology, Schooling and the Family in Postwar Canada.* Toronto: University of Toronto Press, 1999.
- "Disciplining the Student Body: Schooling and the Construction of Canadian Children's Bodies, 1930 to 1960." *History of Education Quarterly* 41, 2 (Summer 2001): 189–215.
- "Race, Class, and Health: School Medical Inspection and 'Healthy' Children in British Columbia, 1890 to 1930." *Canadian Bulletin of Medical History* 19 (2002): 95–112.
- "Between Education and Memory: Health and Childhood in English-Canada, 1900–1945." *Scientia Canadensis* 29, 1 (2006): 49–72.
- Tamara Myers, Leslie Paris, and Veronica Strong-Boag, eds. *Lost Kids: Vulnerable Children and Youth in Twentieth-Century Canada and the United States.* Vancouver: UBC Press, 2010.

Golden, Janet. *Message in a Bottle: The Making of Fetal Alcohol Syndrome.* Cambridge: Harvard University Press, 2005.
- ed. *Infant Asylums and Children's Hospitals: Medical Dilemmas and Developments, 1850–1920.* New York: Garland, 1989.

Goldstein, Tara, and David Selby, eds. *Weaving Connections – Educating for Peace, Social and Environmental Justice.* Toronto: Sumach Press, 2000.

Gould, Stephen J. "Dr. Down's Syndrome." *Natural History* 89, 4 (1980): 142–8.

Gould, Tony. *A Summer Plague: Polio and its Survivors.* New Haven, CT: Yale University Press, 1995.

Haig-Brown, Celia. *Resistance and Renewal: Surviving the Indian Residential School.* Vancouver: Arsenal Pulp Press, 1988.

Halpenny, J., and Lillian Ireland. *How to be Healthy.* Winnipeg and Toronto: W.J. Gage and Company, 1911.

Halpern, Sydney A. *American Pediatrics: The Social Dynamics of Professionalism, 1880–1980.* Berkeley: University of California Press, 1988.

Hayes, Michael T., and Rhonda S. Black. "Troubling Signs: Hollywood Films Movies and the Construction of a Discourse of Pity." *Disability Studies Quarterly* 22, 3 (2003): 114–32.

Heller, Thomas C., Morton Sasna, and David E. Wellbery, eds. *Reconstructing Individualism: Autonomy, Individuality, and the Self in Western Thought.* California: Stanford University Press, 1986.

Hind, Margery. *School House in the Arctic.* London: Geoffrey Bles, 1958.

Holt, L. Emmett. "Health Education of Children." *Canadian Public Health Journal* 13, 3 (March 1922): 104–8.

Holtzman, Neil A., and Robert Haslam. "Elevation of Serum Copper following Copper Sulfate as an Emetic." *Pediatrics* 42, 1 (July 1968): 189–93.

Hoskin, Keith. "The Examination, Disciplinary Power and Rational Schooling." *History of Education* 8, 2 (1979).
Irvine, Janice M. *Talk about Sex: The Battle over Sex Education in the United States*. Berkeley: University of California Press, 2002.
Jeffrey, Jaclyn, and Glenace Edwall, eds. *Memory and History: Essays on Recalling and Interpreting Experience*. Lanham, New York: University Press of America, 1994.
Johnson, F. Henry. *A Brief History of Canadian Education*. Toronto: McGraw-Hill, 1968.
Johnston, Basil. *Indian School Days*. Toronto: Key Porter Books, 1988.
Jones, Andrew, and Leonard Rutman. *In the Children's Aid: J. J. Kelso and Child Welfare in Ontario*. Toronto: University of Toronto Press, 1981.
Jones, Esyllt. *Influenza 1918: Death, Disease, and Struggle in Winnipeg*. Toronto: University of Toronto Press, 2007.
Kelm, Mary-Ellen. *Colonizing Bodies – Aboriginal Health and Healing in British Columbia, 1900–1950*. Vancouver: UBC Press, 1998.
Kendall, Florence P. "Sister Kenny Revisited." *Archives of Physical Medicine and Rehabilitation* 79, 4 (1998): 361–5.
Kerr, M.H. "Defective Children." *Public Health Journal* 6, 12 (December 1915): 618–20.
Kevles, Daniel J. *In the Name of Eugenics: Genetics and the Uses of Human Heredity*. New York: Knopf, 1985.
Key, Ellen. *The Century of the Child*. New York: G.P. Putnam's Sons, 1909.
King, Charles R. *Children's Health in America: A History*. New York: Twayne Publishers, 1993.
Kliewer, Christopher, and Linda May Fitzgerald. "Disability, Schooling and the Artifacts of Colonialism." *Teachers College Record* 103, 3 (June 2001): 450–70.
Knight, A.P. *The Ontario Public School Hygiene*. Toronto: Copp Clark Limited, 1910.
Krohn, William. *First Book in Hygiene – A Primer in Physiology*. New York: D. Appleton and Company, 1907.
Ladd-Taylor, Molly. *Mother-Work: Women, Child Welfare and the State 1890–1930*. Chicago: University of Illinois Press, 1994.
Lambert, Barbara Ann, ed. *Chalkdust and Outhouses – Westcoast Schools, 1893–1950*. Powell River: Barbara Lambert, 2000.
Lee, Annabelle. "Beauty." *Chatelaine* (September 1932.): 26.

Levin, David Michael, and George F. Solomon. "The Discursive Formation of the Body in the History of Medicine." *The Journal of Medicine and Philosophy* 15 (1990): 515–16.
Lewis, Norah. "Creating the Little Machine: Child Rearing in British Columbia, 1919–1939." *BC Studies* 56 (Winter 1982–83): 44–60.
Licht, Sidney, ed. *Therapeutic Electricity and Ultraviolet Radiation*, second edition. New Haven: E. Licht, 1967.
Lim, Sing. *West Coast Chinese Boy*. Montreal: Tundra Books, 1979.
Little, M.J.H. *'No car, no radio, no liquor permit': The Moral Regulation of Single Mothers in Ontario, 1920–1977*. Toronto: Oxford University Press, 1998.
Longmore, Paul and Lauri Umansky, eds. *The New Disability History: American Perspectives*. New York: New York University Press, 2001.
– "The Cultural Framing of Disability: The Telethon as a Case Study." *PMLA* 120, 2 (March 2005): 502–8.
Lucas, C.A. *Public Health Education in the Schools*. British Columbia: Provincial Board of Health, 1926.
Lummis, Jessie I., and Williedell Schawe. *The Safety Hill of Health*. New York: World Book Company, 1927.
MacDougall, Heather. *Activists and Advocates: Toronto's Health Department, 1883–1983*. Toronto: Dundurn Press, 1990.
MacHaffie, Lloyd P. "Pitfalls and Tragedies of the Pre-School Child." *Child and Family Welfare* 12, 1 (May 1936): 9–14.
MacLaren, Angus. *Our Own Master Race: Eugenics in Canada, 1885–1945*. Toronto: University of Toronto Press, 1990.
MacMurchy, Helen. "The Mentally Defective Child." *Public Health Journal* 6, 2 (February 1915): 85–6.
May, Josephine. "Secrets and Lies: Sex Education and the Gendered Memories of Childhood's End in an Australian Provincial City, 1930s to 1950s." *Sex Education* 6, 1 (February 2006): 1–15.
McCullough, John W.S. "Are You Sure of Their Health? An Interesting Challenge to Parents and Teachers Everywhere." *Chatelaine* (December 1930): 9, 57.
McDarmid, Margot. "Native reserves polluted due to gaps in rules: AG." CBC News Online, November 3 2009. *http://www.cbc.ca/canada/story/2009/11/03/vaughan-fraser-auditor-environment-commissioner-report.html* (Retrieved 24 March 2010).
McHenry, E.W. "Nutrition and Child Health." *Canadian Public Health Journal* 33, 4 (April 1942): 54.

McIntosh, J.W. "The Vancouver Outbreak of Haemorrhagic Smallpox II: Lessons Learned from the Outbreak." *Canadian Public Health Journal* 24, 3 (March 1933): 112–19.

McIntosh, Robert. "'Grotesque Faces and Figures': Child Labourers and Coal Mining Technology in Victorian Canada." *Scientia Canadensis* 12, 2 (Fall/Winter 1988): 97–112.

– "Constructing the Child: New Approaches to the History of Childhood in Canada." *Acadiensis* 18, 2 (Spring 1999): 126–40.

– *Boys in the Pit: Child Labour in Coal Mines*. Montreal and Kingston: McGill-Queen's University Press, 2000.

McKendry, J.B.J., and J.D. Bailey. *Paediatrics in Canada*. Ottawa: Canadian Paediatric Society, 1990.

McPhedran, Harris. "The Pre-School Child." *Canadian Medical Association Journal* 20, 6 (June 1929): 658–60.

Meadmore, Daphne. "The Production of Individuality through Examination." *British Journal of Sociology of Education* 14, 1 (1993): 59–73.

Meekosha, Helen, and Leanne Dowse. "Enabling Citizenship: Gender, Disability, and Citizenship in Australia." *Feminist Review* 57 (1997): 49–72.

Miller, J.R. *Shingwauk's Vision – A History of Native Residential Schools*. Toronto: University of Toronto Press, 1996.

Milloy, J.R. *National Crime: Canadian Government and the Residential School System, 1879 to 1976*. Winnipeg: University of Manitoba Press, 1999.

Minnett, Valerie, and Mary-Anne Poutanen. "Swatting Flies for Health: Children and Tuberculosis in Early Twentieth Century Montreal." *Urban History Review* 36: 1 (Fall 2007): 32–60.

Mitchell, David, and Sharon Snyder. "The Eugenic Atlantic: Race, Disability, and the Making of an International Eugenic Science, 1800–1945." *Disability & Society* 18, 7 (December 2003): 843–64.

Mitchell, Duncan, Rannveig Trautadottir, Rohhss Chapman, Louise Townson, Nigel Ingham, and Sue Ledger, eds. *Exploring Experiences of Advocacy by People with Learning Disabilities*. London: Jessica Kingsley Publishers, 2006.

Moffat, Florence C. "Forgotten Villages of the BC Coast – Hospital Life at Bella Bella." *Raincoast Chronicles* 11 (1987): 50–5.

Moffat, Tina, and Ann Herring. "The Historical Roots of High Rates of Infant Death in Aboriginal Communities in Canada in the Early Twentieth Century: The Case of Fisher River, Manitoba." *Social Science and Medicine* 48 (1999): 1821–32.

Moore, Nora. "Child Welfare Work." *The Canadian Nurse* 12, 11 (November 1916): 634–5.

Moore, O.M. "Peptic Ulcers in Children." *Canadian Medical Association Journal* 44, 5 (May 1941): 462–6.

Morgan, George. *Unsettled Places – Aboriginal People and Urbanisation in New South Wales*. Kent Town: Wakefield Press, 2006.

Mundie, G.S. "The Mentally Defective." *Canadian Medical Association Journal* 4, 5 (May 1914): 398.

– "Juvenile Delinquency." *Canadian Medical Association Journal* 5, 5 (May 1915): 405.

Myers, Tamara. "Embodying Delinquency: Boys' Bodies, Sexuality, and Juvenile Justice History in Early Twentieth-Century Quebec." *Journal of the History of Sexuality* 14, 4 (October 2005): 383–414.

– *Caught: Montreal's Modern Girls and the Law, 1869–1945*. Toronto: University of Toronto, 2006.

– and Joan Sangster. "Retorts, Runaways, and Riots: Patterns of Resistance in Canadian Reform Schools for Girls, 1930–1960." *Journal of Social History* 34:3 (Spring 2001): 669–98.

Naylor, C. David, ed. *Canadian Health Care and the State – A Century of Evolution*. Montreal and Kingston: McGill-Queen's University Press, 1992.

Naylor, C. David. *Private Practice, Public Payment: Canadian Medicine and the Politics of Health Insurance, 1911–1966*. Toronto: University of Toronto Press, 1986.

Nichols, Buford L., Angel Ballabriga, and Norman Kretchmer, eds. *History of Pediatrics, 1850–1950*. New York: Raven Press, 1991.

Norcross, Rene. "The Little Brother." *The Canadian Nurse*, II (1915): 436–8.

Olsen, Kent C. *Poisoning and Drug Overdose*. New York: Lang Medical Books/McGraw Hill, 2004.

Olsen, Sylvia. *No Time to Say Goodbye: Children's Stories of Kuper Island Residential School*. Victoria: Sono Nis Press, 2001.

Ouellet, Françoise Miller. "Play Therapy and the Nurse." *The Canadian Nurse* 56, 4 (April 1960): 344–6.

Park, D., and J. Radforth. "From the Case Files: Reconstructing a History of Forced Sterilization." *Disability and Society* 13, 3 (June 1998): 317–42.

Partington, M.W. "Paediatric Admissions to Kingston General Hospital, Kingston Ontario (1899–1909)." *Families* 22, 1 (1983): 33–46.

Paterson, Donald. "Health Services for Handicapped Child in British Columbia." *Canadian Medical Association Journal* 76, 6 (15 March 1957): 483–5.

Pemberton, Kim. "Health officer cites shocking statistics on B.C. child poverty." *Vancouver Sun* (17 June 1998): A1–A2.
Pernick, Martin S. *The Black Stork: Eugenics and the Death of 'Defective' Babies in American Medicine and the Motion Pictures Since 1915.* New York: Oxford University Press, 1996.
Peterson, Alan, and Robin Bunton, ed. *Foucault, Health, and Medicine.* London and New York: Routledge, 1997.
Philmot, B.E.A. "In the Children's Ward." *The Canadian Nurse* 5 (1910): 176–7.
Poutanen, Mary Anne. "Containing and Preventing Contagious Disease: Montreal's Protestant School Board and Tuberculosis, 1900–1947." *Canadian Bulletin of Medical History* 23, 2 (2006): 401–28.
Prescott Munro, Heather. *A Doctor of Their Own: The History of Adolescent Medicine.* Cambridge, MA: Harvard University Press, 1998.
Prout, Alan. *The Future of Childhood – Towards the Interdisciplinary Study of Children.* London and New York: Routledge Farmer, 2005.
Province of British Columbia. *First Report of the Provincial Board of Health.* Victoria: Queen's Printer, 1895.
Read, J., and J. Walmsley. "Historical Perspectives on Special Education, 1890–1970." *Disability & Society* 21, 5 (2006): 455–69.
Robertson, L. Bruce, and Alan Brown. "Blood Transfusion in Infants and Young Children." *Canadian Medical Association Journal* 54 (April 1915): 298–305.
Rooke, Patricia T., and R.L. Schnell. *Discarding the Asylum: From Child Rescue to the Welfare State 1880–1950.* Lanham, MD: University Press of America, 1983.
Ross, John R., and Alan Brown. "Poisonings Common in Children." *Canadian Medical Association Journal* 64, 4 (April 1951): 285–8.
Rutty, Christopher. "The Middle-Class Plague: Epidemic Polio and the Canadian State, 1936–1937." *Canadian Bulletin of Medical History* 13, 2 (1996): 277–314.
– "The Twentieth Century Plague." *The Beaver* 84, 2 (April/May 2004): 32–7.
Ryan, Patrick. "How 'New' is the New Sociology of Childhood: The Myth of a Paradigm Shift." *Journal of Interdisciplinary History* 38, 4 (Spring 2008): 553–76.
Scott, Joan Wallace. "Gender as a Useful Category of Historical Analysis." *American Historical Review* 91, 5 (December 1986): 1053–76.
Shaw, Elizabeth, and Danielle Grenier. "Taking the Pulse of Canadian Children – A Health Report Card for the Millennium." *Paediatric Children Health* 6, 4 (April 2001): 181–3.

Silverthorne, Nelles, Alan Brown, and W.J. Auger. "Pneumonia in Childhood." *Canadian Medical Association Journal* 44, 5 (May 1941): 492–6.
– "Meningitis in Childhood." *Canadian Medical Association Journal* 48, 3 (March 1943): 215–18.
Smith, George E. "The Prevention of Infection in Infancy." *The Public Health Journal* 17, 8 (August, 1926): 405–6.
Snyder, Sharon L., and David T. Mitchell. *Cultural Locations of Disability*. Chicago and London: The University of Chicago Press, 2006.
Standing Senate Committee on Social Affairs, Science and Technology. Report of the Subcommittee on Cities. *In from the Margins: A Call to Action on Poverty, Housing and Homelessness*. Ottawa: Senate Canada, 2009.
Stang, Antonia S., and Arvind Joshi. "The Evolution of Freestanding Children's Hospitals in Canada." *Paediatric Child Health* 11, 8 (October 2006): 501–6.
Statistics Canada, Historical Statistics. "Series B23–34. Average Age Specific Death-Rates, Both Sexes. Canada for five year periods, 1921–1974." http://www.statcan.gc.ca/pub/11-516-x/sectionb/4147437-eng.htm (Retrieved 25 March 2010).
– "Series B59–64. Average Annual Infant Death Rates for Selected Causes, Canada, for Five Year Periods, 1931 to 1974." http://www.statcan.gc.ca/pub/11-516-x/sectionb/4147437-eng.htm#1 (Retrieved 17 February 2012).
Sterling, Shirley. *My Name is Seepeetza*. Toronto: Douglas and McIntyre, 1992.
Stern, Minna Alexandra, and Howard Markel. *Formative Years – Children's Health in the United States, 1880–2000*. Ann Arbor: University of Michigan Press, 2002.
Stevens, W.J. "A Review of Obstetrics." *Canadian Nurse* 23, 9 (September 1927): 465–8.
Stowell, Charles H. *The Essentials of Health. A Text-book on Anatomy, Physiology, and Hygiene*. Toronto: The Educational Book Company, Ltd, 1909.
Strong-Boag, Veronica. "'Today's Child': Preparing for the 'Just Society' One Family at a Time." *Canadian Historical Review* 86, 4 (December 2005): 673–99.
– "'Children of Adversity': Disability and Child Welfare in Canada from the Nineteenth to the Twenty-First Century." *Journal of Family History* 32, 4 (2007): 413–32.
– and Cheryl Krasnick Warsh, eds. *Children's Health Issues in Historical Perspective*. Waterloo: Wilfrid Laurier University, 2005.

Sturrock, John. *The Language of Autobiography – Studies in the First Person Singular*. London: Cambridge University Press, 1993.

Sutherland, Harold. "Health of the Baby Becomes Increasingly Important." *Saturday Night* (23 March 1940): 17.

Sutherland, Neil. *Children in English-Canadian Society: Framing the Twentieth-Century Consensus*. Toronto: University of Toronto Press, 1976.

– "The Triumph of 'Formalism': Elementary Schooling in Vancouver from the 1920s to the 1960s." *BC Studies* 69–70 (1986): 175–210.

Thomson, Gerald. "A Fondness for Charts and Children: Scientific Progressivism in Vancouver Schools 1920 to 1950." *Historical Studies in Education*, 12, 1/2 (2002): 111–28.

– "'Through No Fault of Their Own': Josephine Dauphinee and the 'Subnormal' Pupils of the Vancouver School System, 1911–1941." *Historical Studies in Education* 18, 1 (2006): 51–73.

Thorne, Barrie. "Editorial: Crafting the Interdisciplinary field of Childhood Studies." *Childhood* 14, 2 (May 2007): 149–50.

Tompkins, George. *A Common Countenance: Stability and Change in the Canadian Curriculum*. Scarborough: Prentice Hall, 1986.

Trent, James W. *Inventing the Feeble Mind: A History of Mental Retardation in the United States*. Berkeley: University of California Press, 1994.

University of Toronto. "History of the Department of Paediatrics – Historical Perspectives." *http://www.paeds.utoronto.ca/about/history.htm* (Retrieved 25 March 2010).

Ursel, Jane. *Private Lives, Public Policy: 100 Years of State Intervention in the Family*. Toronto: Women's Press, 1992.

Vertinsky, Patricia. "The Social Construction of the Gendered Body: Exercise and the Exercise of Power." *International Journal of the History of Sport* 11 (August 1994): 147–71.

Vivian, R.P., Charles McMillan, P.E. Moore, E. Chant Robertson, W.H Sebrell, F.F. Tisdall, and W.G. McIntosh. "The Nutrition and Health of the James Bay Indian." *Canadian Medical Association Journal* 59, 6 (December 1948), 505.

Volpe, Peter. "Is Down Syndrome a Modern Disease?" *Perspectives in Biology and Medicine* 29, 3 Part 1 (Spring 1986): 423–36.

Warner, Elizabeth M. "A Survey of Mongolism, with a Review of One Hundred Cases." *Canadian Medical Association Journal* 33, 5 (November 1935): 495–500.

Warren, Olive B. "Rheumatic Fever: Scourge of Childhood." *The Canadian Nurse* 45, 11 (1949): 854–8.

Weisz, George. *Divide and Conquer – A Comparative History of Medical Specialization.* Toronto: Oxford University Press, 2006.

Wharf, Brian, ed. *Community Approaches to Child Welfare.* Toronto: Broadview Press, 2002.

Williams, Robin. *A Vancouver Boyhood – Reflections of Growing up in Vancouver, 1925–1945.* Vancouver: Peanut Butter Publishing, 1997.

Wilson, J.D., Robert M. Stamp, and Louis-Phillippe Audet. *Canadian Education – A History.* Scarborough: Prentice Hall of Canada, Ltd, 1970.

Woods, Pamela J. "Hazardous to Children's Health? New Zealand Primary Schools, 1890–1914." *History News* 66 (1993): 4–7.

Wyllie, J. "Sex Differences in the Mortalities of Childhood and Adult Life." *Canadian Public Health Journal* 24, 11 (November 1933): 530–42.

Young, Judith. "Changing Attitudes Towards Families of Hospitalized Children from 1935 to 1975: A Case Study." *Journal of Advanced Nursing* 17 (1992): 1422–9.

– "'Young Sufferers': Sick Children in Late Nineteenth-Century Toronto." *Nursing History Review* 3 (1995): 129–42.

Zelizer, Viviana A. *Pricing the Priceless Child: The Changing Social Value of Children.* New Jersey: Princeton University Press, 1994.

Index

accidents: in childhood, 4; and death, 10–11, 38; poisoning, 36
adolescence: and gender, 36–8, 50, 65, 133; history of, 6, 9; and medicine, 103
Alberta: and eugenics, 125–8; and health textbooks, 89; and provincial health insurance, 6
Alberta Medical Association, 27, 129
American Pediatric Society, 24

body: doctors' attitudes towards, 29–3; in historical research, 4–5, 7–8, 14, 20
Brankin, David, 123–4
Brown, Alan: and child patients, 31, 33–4; and infant mortality, 24–5, 29, 58, 103
British Columbia: and child poverty, 145; and Department of Neglected Children, 123; and disability in childhood, 8; and First Nations peoples, 43, 100, 105–6; health textbooks in, 37, 68, 87–9, 95–6; and provincial health insurance, 6; and public health, 92; rural schools in, 95

Canadian Medical Association pediatric section, 41
Canadian Mother and Child, The, 28. *See also* Couture, Ernest
Canadian Nursing Association, 38
Canadian Society for the Study of Diseases of Children, 24
chicken pox: control of, 11; in childhood memories, 56, 69, 78, 90
child health centre, 126. *See also* Hastings, Charles
childhood: changing ideology of, 7–9; and child psychology, 93, 134; and children as "not yet adult," 14, 16, 22, 45; diseases of, 31, 69, 110; doctor's attitudes towards, 29–32; and oral history, 6, 15, 143–4; pathologies associated with, 14, 16, 22, 45, 121; in Quebec, 12–3; and race, 42–4; and schooling, 87; and work, 55, 65; and venereal disease, 102, 138

Christianity and health curriculum, 10, 17, 85–9, 93
citizenship: and eugenics, 27; and health, 10, 18, 96–101, 128, 133
class: and attitudes towards health, 24–6, 39–41, 92; as category of historical analysis, 6, 14, 143–4; and eugenic anxieties, 125; and First Nations peoples, 70; in health curriculum, 10, 42, 90, 98–9; and impact on health and welfare, 7, 11, 23, 39; and race, 27
Couture, Ernest, 26–9. See also Canadian Mother and Child, The; Division of Child and Maternal Health

Dauphinee, Josephine, 128
death, 54, 65, 73, 77, 79, 142–3. See also infant mortality
dentist, 57–8, 79, 82. See also teeth
Department of National Health and Welfare, 6
diphtheria: in childhood memories, 51, 54, 77, 105; control of, 11, 29, 67, 90
disability: and "feeble-mindedness," 123–8; intellectual, 121–3; and pedagogy of failure, 19, 121–2, 130, 132–5; physical, 19, 121–2. See also school(ing)
disease: prevention in childhood, 9–12, 17–21, 33–5; and schooling, 86–7, 94
Division of Child and Maternal Health. See Couture, Ernest
doctors: and attitudes towards parents, 25–6, 28; and children's pathology, 30–4; and class, 40–1, 57; and disability, 19, 136; and embodiment of children 12, 16, 126, 143; and eugenic attitudes, 27; and First Nations peoples, 42–4, 89, 138–9; and health curriculum, 89; and knee-high agency, 49, 116; and pediatrics, 12, 16, 21–2, 24, 67; and prevention orientation, 28, 35, 126; and sex education, 71–2; and social services, 109–12
domestic doctoring, 16–8, 23, 91; and fathers, 53; and mothers, 60, 64, 78–84, 91

electrotherapy, 48
eugenics, 27, 123, 125; and health education, 87, 109

First Nations peoples: and assumptions of medical professionals, 42–4; and disability, 123–5; at Fisher River, Manitoba, 42–3; and health effects of colonization, 89–90; oral histories of, 15, 68–77; in patient records, 138–40; and residential schools, 99; and traditional approaches to medicine, 92–3
First World War: and disability, 127–8; and health curriculum, 17, 37, 47, 92
Foucault, Michel, 22, 121
foundling home, 7. See also orphanage

gender: and boys, 37–8, 41, 65, 88; and childhood memories, 17; and citizenship, 5; and disability, 132–3; and girls, 26–8, 50, 63, 65; and health curriculum, 88,

97; and medical treatment, 10, 16; and sexuality, 63, 65, 71
Goutte de lait movement, 8
Great Depression, 5–6, 125; in childhood memories, 58–9, 69–77, 79, 82

Halifax, 91
Hastings, Charles, 126. *See also* child health centre
head lice, 75, 78, 84
health insurance, 6. *See also* Medical Care Insurance Act
heliotherapy, 81
Holt, Emmett, 26–9, 42
home remedies, 22–3; in childhood memories, 4, 58, 60, 78, 80; doctors dismissal of, 23, 51, 91
Hospital for Sick Children (HSC): and Alan Brown, 24; in childhood memories, 4, 59, 72, 107; and patient records, 102, 138. *See also* Toronto
hospitalization: and assumptions about child patients, 115–6; in history of children, 18, 103, 105–6; and nursing, 106–8; and patient visitation, 106–7, 113; and play therapy, 106–8. *See also* nursing

influenza: 1918 pandemic, 6, 47, 91; in childhood memories, 53–4, 110; rates in childhood, 29; and parent medicines, 34
infant mortality: and First Nations peoples, 43; and medical attitudes towards children, 30; and preventative discourse, 26–9, 88, 106; and reduction of, 11, 21–5, 43. *See also* death

Kenny, Elizabeth, 59–60. *See also* poliomyelitis
Key, Ellen, 119
Kingston (Ontario) General Hospital, 50, 105

MacMurchy, Helen, 123–4, 130–1
measles: in childhood memories, 3, 56, 61, 78, 90; and contagious diseases of childhood, 29, 88, 90, 105
Medical Care Insurance Act, 6. *See also* health insurance
Montreal: anti-vaccination riots, 56; Children's Memorial Hospital, 108, 135; and disease prevention, 11; Homeopathic Hospital (Queen Elizabeth Hospital), 57; and infant mortality, 24–5; and pediatric practice, 24; and poverty, 51–3; and religion-affiliated health services, 52, 54–5; Royal Victoria Hospital, 104, 124; Sainte-Justine Hospital, 104, 106; and school truancy, 13
mothers: and domestic doctoring, 3–4, 16–17, 58–60, 75, 78; and eugenics, 27; and hospital birth, 106; and hospital stays, 50; and poverty, 13, 52–3; and professional advice, 23, 31; and professional attitudes towards, 25, 32–4, 110–12, 126; and race, 69–71, 99

nursing, 5; and disease prevention, 25; and First Nations peoples, 43; and play therapy, 106–7. *See also* hospitalization nutrition: in childhood memories, 56–7, 65, 80; and First Nations peoples, 43–4; and gender 38–9; in health curriculum, 17, 85, 100; in infancy, 22, 103; lack of, 26, 76, 105, 145

Ontario Easter Seals, 120
oral history interviews, 5, 15, 19, 86, 141
orphanage, 7, 125. *See also* foundling home

personal hygiene, 41–2
poliomyelitis, 47; and disability, 120, 122; and family coping strategies, 41; and gender, 132–3; and hospitalization, 4, 62–3; and treatment, 48, 51, 56, 59, 81; and schooling, 61, 131. *See also* Kenny, Elizabeth

quarantine, 51, 54–5, 61, 81
Quebec, 8–9
Queen Alexandra Solarium. *See* heliotherapy

race: and attitudes towards health, 26; as a category of historical analysis, 6, 10, 16; and eugenics, 27, 87, 125, 128; and First Nations peoples, 42–4, 83, 139–40; and preventative orientation to health, 41
Regina, 64
rheumatic fever: control of, 36; in patient records, 102, 110–11
Royal College of Physicians and Surgeons of Canada, 67

school(ing): and compulsory attendance, 10; and contagious diseases, 10; as "health laboratories," 9–10; and health lessons, 94, 99, 101; and health textbooks, 17, 37, 98; and nursing, 40, 64, 77, 100; and medical inspection, 9, 35, 67; as unhealthy spaces, 94–5. *See also* disability
Second World War, 11, 67, 82; in childhood memories, 4, 91; and health curriculum, 18, 133–5
sexuality: as a category of historical analysis, 10, 17; and dating, 50–1; and menstruation, 115; and sex education, 71–2
scarlet fever: in childhood memories, 54–6; control of, 29, 40, 88, 105
social work, 5

teeth: advice on brushing, 76; care of, 56–57; extraction of, 17. *See also* water fluoridation
textbooks: and Christian morality, 88–9; and democratic citizenship, 94–7; and disability, 133–4; and gender, 37, 98; and hegemonic health knowledge, 17, 86; and middle-class assumptions, 98; and use in medical schools, 27–9
theory, and size and age as constructed, 12–15, 45
Thistletown Regional Centre, 139
Toronto: and child health centres, 126; and disease prevention, 10; and the growth of pediatrics, 24;

and poverty, 38; and segregation of "defective" children, 123, 130. *See also* Hospital for Sick Children (HSC)
tuberculosis: in childhood memories, 54, 81; control of, 11, 27, 35, 38, 125

vaccination: in childhood memories, 39, 56, 85; and controversy, 9, 67; and disease prevention, 10
Vancouver: and classes for "subnormal" students, 128-9; and traditional Chinese medicine, 93

Vancouver General Hospital, 33, 49

wars. *See* First World War; Second World War
water fluoridation, 9, 67
welfare state, 5-7, 12-3
whooping cough: in childhood memories, 78, 91; control of, 11, 29, 90;
Winnipeg, 25, 38; influenza pandemic of 1918, 6, 54